Group Experience as a Resource

Volker Münch

Group Experience as a Resource

Invitation to a Change of Perspective in Group Psychotherapy and Self-Experience

Springer

Volker Münch
Psychologische Praxis
München, Germany

ISBN 978-3-662-70866-8 ISBN 978-3-662-70864-4 (eBook)
https://doi.org/10.1007/978-3-662-70864-4

This book is a translation of the original German edition "Gruppenerleben als Ressource" by Volker Münch, published by Springer-Verlag GmbH, DE in 2024. The translation was done with the help of an artificial intelligence machine translation tool. A subsequent human revision was done primarily in terms of content, so that the book will read stylistically differently from a conventional translation. Springer Nature works continuously to further the development of tools for the production of books and on the related technologies to support the authors.

This Springer imprint is published by the registered company Springer-Verlag GmbH, DE, part of Springer Nature.
The registered company address is: Heidelberger Platz 3, 14197 Berlin, Germany

Preface and Acknowledgements

The experience of being part of a group in one's own life is an important factor for a person who works psychotherapeutically. It can be helpful not only in the context of their group work, but also when it comes to relating people in individual therapy more to contact with other people. Negative experiences with groups, especially in the first important group, the primary family, are often crucial in the development of depressions and anxiety disorders, compulsions and personality accentuations. Good group experiences, on the other hand, carry the individual through difficult times and represent a resource, internally as well as in external reality.

Farhad Dalal, in his book *Taking the group seriously*, already pointed out at the end of the 1990s that, in his opinion, there needed to be a paradigm shift in the way groups should be understood and how work should be done in groups. Our view of humans as beings separated from their environment and others, which stems from individual treatment, too quickly forgets, in his opinion, that the human psyche should always be thought of as connected with the groups in which it lives. The so-called intersubjective turn in psychoanalysis has already taught us that any attempt to think of mental suffering as separate from its environment must be considered inadequate. Any treatment approaches, including those in groups, should be guided by this. Both the current societal disruptions and division processes, as well as the increasingly apparent consequences of our human interaction with the natural environment, indicate that we should learn to think more systemically and complexly. This also applies to the models of our own coexistence. The thinking of humans as isolated beings is thus, unsurprisingly, in line with one-sided societal notions and ideologies of self-determination and autonomy, as can also be found in the neoliberal image of humans. Corrections are needed here, which also affect the work of psychotherapists.

What are Groups?

Groups are a peculiar phenomenon. There are theorists who assume that groups are always just a mental event. Groups as such may not exist, at least not in the way we imagine them in light of the individuals who come together to form a group. Groups are always more than the sum of their participants, they breathe a spirit, they have a unique character. Groups and group experiences are initially an idea, something abstract and yet at the same time something experiential and tangible. Why is that? Perhaps it could be formulated in such a way that groups allow one to participate in the greater whole to which we are connected. Thus, groups also have a transcendent, a transpersonal, and even a spiritual dimension. In groups, one can experience the unusual and the transcendent, groups are then very real in psychological perception and they have a lasting influence on our feeling for whether and where we have a place in the world and whether we can feel at home in it.

The Experience of Connectedness

In the context of this experience of connectedness, we can also draw on related inner resources in the face of difficulties. These resources are not only the "property" of the individual, but of people in general, and in turn refer to others in various group contexts. In other words: The image of others in me is crucial to whether and how I find myself. This book will revolve around this thought again and again. And it will be about to what extent group experience represents a "treasure" for psychotherapy, but not only in relation to psychotherapy itself. Group therapy can also have a societal function of its own.

I must apologize to all child and adolescent psychotherapists. Since I myself have neither theoretical nor practical experience with groups of children or adolescents, I unfortunately have to abstain from this topic. Since I go into more detail on these life phases in the first part of the book, some of the conclusions I reach can certainly also be applied to this work. Groups with children and adolescents require even more of what I consider necessary for adult therapists, namely personal creativity, flexibility, and commitment.

I thank all the people who have helped me gather challenging and helpful group experiences: Inge Hallmann-Daum and Ulrich Stuck, for introducing me to the human group entity in very different ways, but each very sustainably. My patients, who challenge me in my groups, gift me, and continually teach me new things. My colleagues in the supervision groups, in the MAP group lecturer team, and in the DGAP group forum, who enrich, stimulate, and criticize me. I also thank my colleagues Claudine Schauer, Joachim Weimer, and Sebastian Kudritzki, who have thoroughly co-read parts of the manuscript. Finally, my partner, who knew how to integrate the group thing so naturally into herself and also into our shared life, that our circle of friends today is largely a common and shared one and thus conversely an important aspect of our relationship. Finally, special thanks go to Monika Radecki from Springer-Verlag, who, as in the past, always accompanied me gently and at the same time motivatingly with this group book. The same thanks go to Rahul Ravindran and Omika Mohan, who have professionally and always friendly advanced the production process.

Munich
in March 2024

Volker Münch

Contents

About the Author

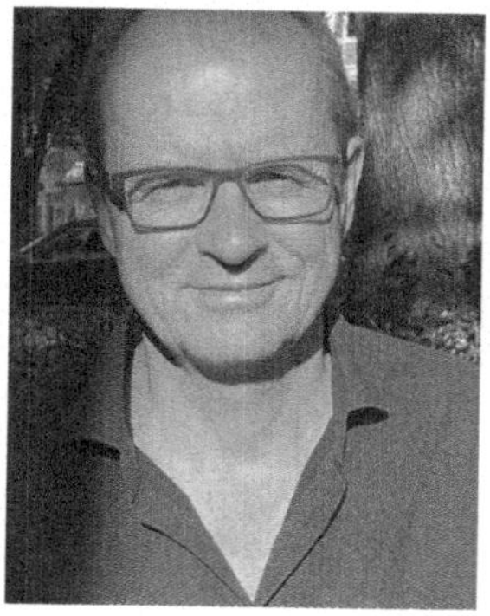

Dipl. Psych. Volker Münch, Psychological psychotherapist in private practice in Munich. Individual and group analyst. Individual and group teaching analyst, -supervisor and lecturer at the MAP, Munich. Balint group leader. KBV expert. Publications on the topics of therapeutic attitude, digitalization, midlife crisis, culture and society.

Introduction 1

Abstract

The topic of groups and group psychotherapy is introduced. Why is there too little group therapy? What connections to society and our socialization exist in understanding our reluctance towards group phenomena? Why are these fears primarily associated with loss of self and regression? It turns out that an individual cannot be well understood without their integration or lack of integration into groups. Finally, groups have an ethical aspect: they enable transparency and counteract ethically unacceptable behavior by individuals in positions of power.

1.1 Our Life in Groups

This book is about experiencing life in groups. This experience in groups is ultimately an experience of ourselves as part of groups. This is an important point: Because if individuals are thought of as separate from the processes in the groups surrounding them, we cannot adequately account for the constitution of our psyche. According to the latest concepts, we cannot be thought of as separate from the structures in which we move and in which we grow up. We develop in groups and at the same time despite these groups, by taking a different developmental path each time. The resources, the raw material for this psychological development, we largely derive from our culture, our environment, from contact with the people who are important to us.

This has political implications. A view of humanity that is accustomed to thinking of one person as completely separate from another, of humans as separate from nature, and, underlying this, of mind from matter, does not nearly describe the world in which we live, according to current research and measured by the

V. Münch, *Group Experience as a Resource*,
https://doi.org/10.1007/978-3-662-70864-4_1

devastation caused by this worldview. Our incomplete and one-sidedly autonomy-emphasizing view of humanity is thus revealed in our dealings with other people and with the world as such. The hypertrophy of the views of the Western world in the last centuries decisively points to the fact that we have thought and felt ourselves too little as connected, as too little in groups and too little as participants in something greater, and have accordingly acted inappropriately. The bill for this is now to be paid: Wars and crises such as the climate crisis can also be interpreted as a return of this repressed. Artistic productions such as films can also illustrate this. The mega-success "Avatar" (Cameron, 2009) and its planned sequels, for example, address exactly this torn bond between technology-loving humanity (there the "sky people") and the native Navi, perhaps an abbreviation for "native people". While human culture seems to know only subjugation and exploitation, the world of the Navi is characterized by harmony of life with the surrounding nature.

Groups and Emotions

We all try to share our feelings in groups, to communicate them and to find resonance. In the best case, we experience that other people seem to feel very similar to us, and we begin to experience and thus to believe that we are not alone with our inner, personal experiences. This can help to validate our own inner world and also to gradually structure it and thus better understand it. But this increases our social competence. When we join groups, this emotional note can also lead us to take more extreme positions if we seem to be closer to others as a result. An extreme opinion or an extremely strong feeling are much easier to accept than contradictory, multi-layered feelings. Here, it is first and foremost about self-acceptance, about the acceptance of feelings in ourselves, by ourselves. Shared emotions are the strongest social bond and not to be underestimated, as they can be associated with great feelings of satisfaction and also happiness. Therapeutic groups try to combine both: the group experience of shared emotions and the experience of the individual in the group, to remain a part of a group despite differing, differently sounding opinions. Here, the full range of seemingly contradictory human needs for autonomy on the one hand and for belonging on the other can unfold and show itself.

If not enough good group experiences could be collected, not even in the primary group of the family of origin, then groups are often avoided and devalued. Or groups are used so strongly for the creation of an identity that they are virtually abused for this purpose. Then the "others" actually have no real chance to be seen. So there are certainly many "groups" without real, reciprocal contact and probably even more often groups without any reflection on the conditions of their existence. They are then simply taken for granted and the group identity is used as a kind of "filling" to compensate for profound personal insecurities. We will come to the topic of emotions and group at many points, indirectly and also in its special consequences.

The Boy Needs Fresh Air
Another film addresses the interconnectedness of people, especially in the context of the aftermath of war and depression. At the end of the film adaptation of his autobiographical novel *The Boy Needs Fresh Air* (Link, 2018), the author, Hape Kerkeling, himself talks about the people who have accompanied him on his life's journey. They are a part of him, he is them: Kerkeling continues: "It took a while for me to understand. This is all that I am. I am my mother, my father, my brother, and my grandparents. I am their laughter and their pain. I am Aunt Gertrud, Aunt Annemarie and Aunt Veronika, Aunt Lisbeth and Uncle Kurt. I am Mrs. Rädecker and Mrs. Strecker. I am the direction in which my mother pushed me in the pram. I am the spotted cow in the pasture, the yellow grain in the field, and the red poppy by the wayside. I am the cloudless sky. I am awake."

At the end of the scene, which shows the young Hans-Peter with his relatives on their way to a picnic, the adult Kerkeling looks back at the group and his former self. It is deeply touching how the scene and the poetic text express both the connection with the important and formative people in life, with all their good and bad sides, and how helpful it can be for us to transport ourselves back into our early history. This is exactly what happens in psychotherapies. Kerkeling presents himself as someone who has not lost contact with his childlike self, but can see in it a source of creativity and humor, especially because it is also not a simple childhood in post-war Germany.

We will later address individual aspects of what is presented here in a highly condensed form, such as the currently discussed "inner groupality" of humans and C. G. Jung's idea of the "dissociability of the psyche" and much more. These ideas, which are becoming increasingly important in the field of psychotherapy, indicate how important it is for people to recognize their connection with other people, to experience it and to draw from it, in order to better cope with the increasingly complex everyday life. Group psychotherapy and analysis are the royal road to this realization: The experience of connectedness (see also Jaenicke 2006) is one of the most important factors in psychotherapies. The "life-giving" (cf. Symington 1999) encounter with the other and others in the context of therapy and of course also in everyday life can counteract narcissistic, depressive symptoms and other limitations and promote psychological flexibility, stability and balance. And of course, humor is always needed for this.

1.2 Life is a Group Event

From the beginning, we are not alone. Not only do we all come from our mother's body, where we, conceived by our father, were able to grow for about nine months. Kim de l'Horizon has poetically explored in his award-winning *Blood Book*(2022) the different origins we can simultaneously carry within us and how confusing, but also enriching, this can be. It always starts with people who want to have children, to have offspring. Our parents had the same fate, they come from their parents, who come from their parents, in the end the family trees of the individual fan out more and more. We are mentally and often unconsciously deeply shaped by our ancestors, by their desires, hopes and fears. All these people have shaped us, without them we would not be who we are. The illusion of absolute separation, as it has entered our concept of autonomy and independence, is questioned in such moments and the psyche becomes permeable.

I want to emphasize that my concern is to give greater weight to the idea of the group in psychotherapy and analysis. I do not want to question the meaningfulness and successes of individual psychotherapy across the board. Since Analytical Psychology in our context, following C. G. Jung, early fell under suspicion of sympathy with mass movements and regressive currents, my aim is to show that sometimes it is precisely the neglect of the collective in favor of particular interests that leads to the destructive forces expressed in groups breaking through again and again. Individuals do not need to position themselves *against* groups to assert themselves. They even gain strength when they remain sufficiently aware of their inner connection with others, including certain affiliations with groups.

Boundary Issues

Most neurotic disorders are boundary issues. Difficulties in setting boundaries, overstepping, inability to say no, and various forms of sensitivity are cardinal symptoms in the practices of psychotherapists. This shows that it is not only in human nature to want to experience and see oneself as independent from others, but often there is also an immensely strong desire to belong, to feel connected, or even to merge. This, in view of the human condition, our physical separateness, must repeatedly fail, but nonetheless drives us to try it in new ways and again and again. Boundaries are important for building a sense of coherence and identity. However, excessive interest in boundary drawing can prevent one from really letting other people get close, empathizing, being impressed, learning from them.

Especially in therapeutic groups, people learn both: to set boundaries and—once they have staked out enough of their own territory—to engage, to trust, even to love. Without these securities, we have too much to lose. Anyone who puts all their eggs in one basket and expects the world from their partner will inevitably be disappointed. At the same time, we are still more than our connections to others. We are what we bring into the world. Differences in temperament, for example, belong here, as do talents, abilities, weaknesses, vulnerabilities, what we have learned to see as strengths and weaknesses. Our psychological development is thought in C. G. Jung's Analytical Psychology in such a way that it is not only the biography that leaves its traces, but that we process biographical experiences in different ways, depending on who we are. Here the archetypal dimension of the human psyche comes into play. More on this later.

The Psychological Legacy of Ancestors

The behavior of our ancestors can quite profanely express itself in us by carrying their psychological burden, their inhibitions and fears, but also their pleasure and talents within us. Be it that they were biologically inherited to us, be it that they were psychologically conveyed to us through the transgenerational transmission of psychological content—without words, speechless, implicitly through their behavior, non-behavior, speechlessness and (un)noticeable omissions in the biographies, which often point to traumatic experiences. The fact that human experience is shareable always also means that it is not only unique, but also nothing completely new. We live in this contradiction. We have learned, especially in times of increasing individualism, to understand ourselves as separate, autonomous, and independent and to strive to be as little dependent on others as possible. The denial of the other pole of this experience, namely the fact of our participation in what all people share, then our deep dependence on the love of other people, and, as seems to become apparent to us very late, also on the functioning of a healthy natural environment, is involved in the emergence of a multitude of current problems and this applies to the personal, societal and ultimately global level. The illusion of independence, even to its narcissistic extreme form, the idea of immortality, has led to epidemic problems such as addictions, mental disorders, withdrawal, technicism in dealing with each other, contempt for feelings and a false importance of vulnerabilities. Daniele Giglioli has collected interesting thoughts on this in *The Victim Trap* (2015). Wolfgang Schmidbauer (2023) discusses a different approach to dealing with narcissistic patients. The often discussed, but in my opinion overestimated societal tendency to divide also means that we can no longer deal with ourselves and others in a healthy way. The assumption of changing group identities and the respective fight against the "others" seem helpless, as groups are no longer really perceived as helpful, nourishing and supportive units of social cohesion, but rather as combat groups. The fact that there is such a thing as cultural identity is also doubted from a social philosophical perspective (cf. Jullien 2017). So we try to find support in group identities on the net, for example, but overlook the fact that the connections within these groups can only be superficial and not supportive.

People Always Live in Groups

Our entire Western thinking has not only promoted the separation of mind and body since the Enlightenment and made us believe that we could ultimately function perfectly like machines. A second false idea is added: that of man as a being who can live without groups. Group phenomena were long dismissed in psychology and psychotherapy as less important, as primitive, as "mass psychology". The fact that groups have secured our survival in our history, that we could do nothing and are nobody except as part of groups, is not appreciated in this world of the idea of neatly separated individual beings. Even the American psychiatrist Robert Waldinger (2023), who leads long-term studies on the topic of "happiness", comes to the conclusion: "The key to a good life is relationships." And he states: "In our study, we generally found that people are happier when they deal with things that go beyond the self." So there are very definite indications of the importance of contact with other people in our lives.

1.3 Group Therapy and Ethics

The aforementioned deficiency is evident in the marginality of group therapy in Germany, even in the field of psychodynamic psychotherapies. After a boom in the 1960s and 1970s, the vast majority of psychotherapies conducted in Germany were individual therapies. The dangers and risks of this setting, in addition to its significant possibilities, only came to consciousness late (cf. Löwer-Hirsch 2017; Schleu 2012). The question arises whether and if so, how group psychotherapy helps to prevent boundary violations. After all, there are always "witnesses" to the interventions that psychotherapists use there. Or are there also "dangers" in group psychotherapies of behaving erroneously or even harmfully as a psychotherapist?

Example

Once, when I allowed myself to be carried away to interpret to a patient, who provoked impatience and anger in the countertransference, that if she was constantly dissatisfied with her income, she would have to look for a new job, I was plagued by remorse afterwards. I apologized to her, who did not find this intervention in the group as offensive. The other group members took over the criticism of me, telling me that my reaction had been "quite harsh". ◄

In the meantime, through the work of ombudsmen and ethics committees in therapeutic training institutions and professional associations, improved transparency and many insights into the conditions that seemed to have favored such misconduct up to criminal offenses have developed, in addition to shocking insights into derailed treatments. However, this also shows the effectiveness of groups that reflect on group work: The triangulating and controlling function of committees in ethics work and the awareness of being embedded in collegial networks can help to heal and prevent further avoidable misconduct.

As an ethical challenge in a much larger context, we must say goodbye to cherished certainties that suggest that we can continue to live our lives as individuals undisturbed in the face of global issues that confront us all as a crisis. The retreat into a life of prosperity and consumption will work less and less. Ever new groups of people are becoming more visible and articulate their discontent about the conditions, about unfair trade and increasing ecological and climatic unreasonableness. Migrants come to us in large numbers. Many in Western societies seem to have lost their sense of community, the joy of shared experiences, the participation in solidarity. However, world history seems to want to pull us away from the domestic fireplace and ask us where our place is. We must ask ourselves which groups we feel we belong to, who would help us in need, who we really trust and who we love.

The Longing for Paradise

Many patients are used to coping with their lives alone and wanting to do everything without help, so they usually decline gratefully when I suggest group therapy to them. It appears to them as a loss of the intimacy of an exclusive dyadic relationship. In the groups, on the other hand, they believe it is about the supposedly "others" who make their own problems even more unbearable with their problems, those who "talk too much", no, they definitely want individual therapy. Understandable for people with a difficult biography: One would like to go back to childhood and have the "good" mother all to oneself. One would prefer to "return to paradise" (cf. Jacobi 1980).

1.4 The Matrix

But who is this individual, if not a node in a network of relationships? This is how S. Foulkes (1974), considered one of the founders of group therapy, saw the matrix, the groups that they represent, that they are. Like the patients, the therapists are also embedded in networks, in groups, in shared experiences with other people, which are often deeply internalized and strongly shape new relationships. Even if only two people are present in the treatment room, psychologically there are always several people, even groups of people, "virtually" in the room and not only those who are actively talked about. The fact that every person brings their previous group experiences into encounters with people may be a banal insight. And yet, so far there are few concepts of how to imagine this "social unconscious", as Foulkes has formulated it. Even in group therapies, there is sometimes a tendency to continue to individualize problems, to focus on individual participants and to apply the same concepts as in individual treatment. Dalal (1998) also complains about Foulkes' own focus on biographical, psychodynamic aspects of the group participants: "The point this discussion is to show the remarkable absence of the use of the here-and-now, as well as the absence of the social, by Foulkes and Anthony." (ibid., p. 73). Nevertheless, Foulkes wrote elsewhere: "Group-analytic psychotherapy … is neither psychoanalysis of the individuals in the group nor is it the psychoanalytic treatment of a group by a psychoanalyst. It is a kind of psychotherapy of the group by the group, including its leader." (Foulkes 1978, cf. Stuck 2016, p. 78).

This corresponds to a common observation that can be made as a psychotherapist: Often it only becomes apparent in a group how a person really lives with other people, how he reacts, what he or she says and also what not, especially when comparing this behavior with that in the individual setting.

Example

When I admitted a patient, who was now in the middle of life, into one of my groups after a long individual therapy, he had a particularly hard time at the beginning. His inability to connect with others, to really feel something positive, became overly clear. His deep despair and anger also became more apparent than in individual treatment. However, others reacted to him and gradually mutual interest and more differentiated relationships developed in the group context. The relationship with me also gradually changed and became more reconciled. The triangulating and calming effect of the group began to reach him. ◄

1.5 Society *in* the Individual

The fact that people come from different social backgrounds and social strata, that they have internalized their experiences with societal structures, which often have sexist, racist, and colonialist backgrounds in which the individuals and their ancestors were either victims or perpetrators, sometimes both, is currently receiving more societal attention. The focus on the pathology of the individual, which can always be understood as suffering from the ways a society deals with these initially different, resistant individuals, often overlooks this dynamic. Criticism of society has become rare in the field of psychotherapy, as if one did not want to spoil it in the identification with a system that has provided one with prosperity as a psychotherapist. Who would saw off the branch he is sitting on? (cf. Münch 2021).

The reports from psychotherapies are increasingly similar. In ever new variations, the often early deprivations of patients are described, who have to deal with overwhelmed mothers and fathers absent for various reasons. In the search for recognition, mirroring, and love, disappointment, resentment, and despair, neurotic attempts at relationships, and somatizations are constantly being created anew. The accumulation of certain symptoms in certain historical epochs or in certain social milieus clearly points to the influence of overarching forces affecting larger societal milieus, which would require an understanding of group dynamics that allow and make this possible. In group therapies, patients usually notice the opposite, contrary to their primary expectation mentioned above, that they receive added value there, which can hardly be named or even quantified in the currency of dyadic exchange. Groups are and offer more than the sum of their participants, this can hardly be described, but can only be personally experienced. They offer the experience of the "group". In this book, we want to ask what could be at work here.

Ego Work In Action

Viewed from a completely different perspective, namely that of the analysis of the individual personality, the integration into groups can not only be described externally. Not only has every person made a multitude of group experiences and these have, mostly unconsciously, flowed into personal development. The inner constitution of the individual can also be understood as a kind of inner group. We are always already many, in the sense of the book title by Richard David Precht (2009). C. G. Jung already spoke of the "dissociability of the psyche" (cf. Meier 2017), of its multilayeredness and multifacetedness. Most recently, the psychoanalyst R. Kaes spoke of the "inner groupality" (2009) of every human being. This is also the prerequisite for the effect of groups on us. In these, we find in the external different expressions and forms of expression for our various inner parts. Foulkes spoke of group experience and group work as "ego work in action" and I think this image captures well that the mirroring and limitation by others, the possibility of identification and empathy with others, significantly determine the self-feeling and can thus also change it. The idea of an individual existing independently of others is a mental construct and not insignificantly due to the still prevailing image of the enlightened human being as an independent being guided solely by his reason. For Foulkes and today's group analysts, rather, *the group* is at the beginning of every psychological development and also the analysis of the individual. From their imprints and structures, different individual beings and characters develop. With Donald Winnicott (1970), the well-known British child psychiatrist who once said: "There is no such thing as an infant", and who wanted to highlight the mutual dependence of the mother-child system, one could, applied to the group theme, say that there is no individual without a group, and of course, this is more obvious to us, no group without individuals.

Combination Therapy
Both experiences, that of individual as well as group therapy, prove to be significant and indispensable for many patients: allowing closeness in a dyadic relationship, but also opening up and setting boundaries in a group. One can hardly dare to do one without the other, because both require the courage to face one or more others. But this requires a certain degree of inner security and confidence. Therefore, it is often more difficult for more severely affected people to benefit from groups. If traumatic experiences were made in the primary group, i.e., the family, then it is extraordinarily difficult to gain trust and to feel, accept, and use what groups are capable of giving for one's own growth. This often requires prior or parallel individual therapy. We will return to this so-called combination therapy in the second part of the book.

1.6 The Structure of the Book

This book will be less a collection of treatment vignettes and not a presentation of the problems of specialized groups, such as in a clinical context or against the background of certain diseases. Certainly, these topics will be touched upon at some point, but mostly to illustrate which active moments can be observed in group work. My aim is to explore the concept of the group itself and relate it to human biography and becoming a human being in society, to emphasize more than has usually been shown how much we are group beings at our core. Beyond this insight, often sold as banality because it is not really understood and penetrated, it should become clear through many everyday and treatment vignettes what is meant by this. If these facts were better known, we would see a greater spread of group therapy than in recent times. There are signs that something is changing. C. Schöps (2023) pointed out once again in the *ZEIT* that this could also add an important building block to the misery of the care of mentally ill people, if more practitioners offered group therapies.

Each reader should be taken on a journey into their own group biography in this way. This is accompanied by an invitation to reflect on how oneself and of course also today's individual and group patients are shaped by these internalized group experiences. We will understand that societal and cultural phenomena, and thus also zeitgeist phenomena, shape our group identity. In this respect, this book is both in terms of its motivation and background as well as its conception a professional book that wants to remind us sustainably of the personal anchors of our professional therapeutic identity and may help us to open up further to the group idea. Especially when the obvious is not obviously present and given, a sensitivity for the importance of the topic develops. Especially when one can say what happens when the experience of group reference and connection to fellow human beings is questioned or missing, it becomes all the more deeply tangible in contrast what it can mean and how healing it is to feel connected to groups, to others. Ultimately, it means being able to feel truly connected with oneself only then.

The First Part of the Book

In the first part of the book, we will proceed based on the characteristic features and phases in the human life cycle and describe the respective supportive or inhibiting and problematic group experiences of the different ages. As we will see, group experiences typically build on each other and can thus also mutually enrich each other. Missing experiences, on the other hand, lead to isolation, withdrawal, and narcissism. We will have to discuss this latter development as a paradigmatic contrast to healthy development within groups.

The Second Part of the Book

In the second part of the book, we will get to know the various forms of application of depth psychology-based and analytical group psychotherapy, as practiced and represented by the author mainly within the framework of Analytical Psychology. It is also about the possibilities of applying individual and group therapy together in the German statutory health insurance system today. The ideas of Jung's Analytical Psychology and his successors, but also of the Britons Nitsun (2014) and Dalal will occupy us. It will become clear that a comprehensive theory of group practice is not yet available. This contrasts sharply with the vast corpus of knowledge in individual treatment. This is particularly regrettable, as understanding also collective societal processes would depend crucially on us having more knowledge here and applying the existing knowledge.

City Groups

A positive example of this application of group-analytical know-how in new contexts are the open discussion circles, such as the "city group" founded in Munich by Beate Bever-Goldbrich, Mandy Koplin, Magdalena Lechner, Rudolf Tauscher and Adrienn Weiß, a format that is now also being established in other places by committed and concerned psychotherapists at their places of residence.

In these, citizens of various origins should be able to enter into conversation with each other without evaluating or even attacking each other. Topics chosen are conflict-ridden contents such as gendering, financial distress, migration and so on. The background is the long-observed tendency of certain sections of the population to feel socially disadvantaged and not heard by an academic class titled as "elite" and the often resulting dynamics of division and projection. In these contexts too, group-analytical, group-therapeutic knowledge can be made available to the general public in a beneficial way.

In accordance with my broad spectrum, I will mostly use the terms group psychotherapy and group analysis as well as analytical group psychotherapy as an application in the German statutory health insurance system and ultimately also my orientation in group work in the tradition of Jung's Analytical Psychology synonymously. I want to express that it is about the people who treat and those who are treated, and theories often play a subordinate role in practice. Rather, it is about flexibility, creativity, humor, authenticity and the never-ending effort to understand the psychodynamics presented to us.

References

Cameron, J (2009) Avatar—Aufbruch nach Pandora. Film

Dalal, F (1998) Taking the group seriously. Jessica Kingsley Publishers, London

De l'Horizon, K (2022) Blutbuch. Dumont, Köln

Foulkes, S (1974) Gruppenanalytische Psychotherapie. Klotz, Neulingen

Giglioni, D (2015) Die Opferfalle. Matthes und Seitz, Berlin

Jacobi, M (1980) Sehnsucht nach dem Paradies. Bonz, Stuttgart

Jaenicke, C (2006) Das Risiko der Verbundenheit. Klett-Cotta, Stuttgart

Jullien, F (2017) Es gibt keine kulturelle Identität. Suhrkamp, Berlin

Kaes, R (2009) Innere Gruppen und psychische Gruppalität: Entstehung und Hintergründe eines Konzepts. Psyche, 2009, 63(3), 281–305. Klett-Cotta, Stuttgart

Link, C (2018) Der Junge muss an die frische Luft. Verfilmung von H. Kerkelings Buch

Löwer-Hirsch, M (2017) Sexueller Missbrauch in der Psychotherapie. Psychosozial-Verlag, Gießen

Meier, I (2017) Komplexe und Dissoziationen. Brandes und Apsel Verlag, Frankfurt/M

Münch, V (2021) Die therapeutische Haltung. Kohlhammer, Stuttgart

Nitsun, M (2014) The Anti-Group. Routledge, London

Precht, R D (2009) Wer bin ich und wenn ja, wie viele? Pinguin Random House Verlagsgruppe GmbH, München

Schleu, A (2012) Umgang mit Grenzverletzungen. Springer, Berlin

Schmidbauer, W (2023) Facetten und Entwicklungen des Narzissmus-Konzepts. Quelle: https://wolfgang-schmidbauer.de/wp-content/uploads/2013/05/Facetten_Narzissmuss.pdf (Stand: 27.08.2023)

Schöps, C (2023) Mut zur Gruppe. ZEIT 6, 7.3.2023: https://www.zeit.de/2023/06/therapieplatz-psychotherapie-wartezeiten-depressionen-gruppentherapie. (Stand: 3.2.2023)

Stadtgruppe München im Kulturzentrum Luise: https://www.luise-kultur.de/termine/stadt-gruppe/05-05-23. (Stand: 1.9.2023)

Stuck, U (2016). Plädoyer für den Gruppengedanken in der Analytischen Psychologie. In: Schimkus M, Stuck U (Eds) Selbst, Ich und Wir. Brandes und Apsel Verlag, Frankfurt/M

Symington, N (1999) Narzissmus. Psychosozial-Verlag, Gießen

Winnicott, D W (1970) The Maturational Processes and the Facilitating Environment. Karnac, London

Waldinger, R (2023) Wie wird man glücklich? Interview mit M. Stäuble, 19.1.2023 in der SZ-online. Quelle: https://www.sueddeutsche.de/projekte/artikel/gesellschaft/glueck-beziehungen-robert-waldinger-e276198/?reduced=true. (Stand: 22.4.2023)

Part I
Mental Development as a Group Event

The Social Nature of Humans and the New Media

2

Abstract

This chapter aims to investigate the influence of social media usage on group formation and the role of group experiences and group self-experience. Many of us spend hours in the virtual group contexts of social media today. The complex interplay of virtual and real group experiences is still very little researched. Critical perspectives often dominate, but they must remain incomplete and one-sided as long as they make theory-guided assumptions the prerequisite for their considerations.

The exclusive view of psychotherapists on individuals is too short-sighted. Elias (1994) and Dalal (1998) also make it clear: If the individual is seen as influenced by groups, that is, only from the outside, this is too short-sighted. For them, it is not about the influence of the individual on the group, nor about the reverse direction of effect, nor finally about an interaction between outside and inside, but outside and inside are inappropriate concepts for understanding psychological reality. The dichotomies mentioned prove to be problematic as they generate a thinking in opposites, which does not do justice to the real dynamics. Our identity is so much that of a group member, a participant, that we cannot assume that individuals can ever be thought of as independent of the social. The artificial assumption that there is *one* psychological reality in the individual before a group and others influence him, is statically thought and is a thinking in monads. One could rather speak of the fact that we are born into the psyche of a group, so to speak. It is difficult to become aware of this way of thinking and especially its consequences. We are all very influenced by cause-and-effect thinking, which always thinks in vectors, in terms such as me and you, here and there, now and then. To understand the dimension of change in our interaction, as brought about by social media, it may be useful to move away from outdated, simplifying views and try with Dalal (1998) to

V. Münch, *Group Experience as a Resource*,
https://doi.org/10.1007/978-3-662-70864-4_2

develop an understanding of group processes that can be derived from the respective functioning of groups and their group dynamics.

Are groups less attractive today?
My colleague Ulrich Stuck recently reminded in a personal communication that the "pull" into groups, primarily self-experience groups, noticeable in the 1960s and 1970s, has significantly decreased. When people seek psychotherapy, they no longer primarily think of participating in a group, but are usually motivated to do so by us therapists. Occasionally, patients have had good experiences with groups in psychosomatic clinics and then one can assume a better motivation for participation in outpatient groups. In general, however, persuasion is required. Few group participants regret their decision for the group afterwards, many show high appreciation for the experiences made and the changes experienced in their perception and behavior. We will later discuss the influences of the increasingly narcissistic society on the psychological development of individuals. However, the colleague mentioned above is primarily concerned with the impression that we should try to rethink group experience more comprehensively and anew in view of the multitude of virtual contacts, of social groups on the net, of the increasingly extensive and faster and above all increasingly self-evident exchange on these levels. I would like to join this impression.

The experience in virtual contacts and groups has definitely gained influence on the well-being and inner belonging of many people. It would be necessary to ask how these non-physically present groups could gain such importance. Also to what extent the restrictions of exchange on the net influence and possibly impair the perception of the live group on site. The keyword networking is on everyone's lips, my colleagues Altmeyer and Kächele (2006) tried almost 20 years ago to describe what the paradigm shift towards intersubjective viewing means for psychoanalysis. Meanwhile, this perspective has largely prevailed in therapeutic work. At the same time, however, everyday life and the technical changes made in it have become much more complex and multi-layered. All the more, in view of the spread of social media, especially among younger people, the question must be asked what influences can be observed on the formation of psychological structures. One does not have to be as pessimistic as Türcke (2012) or Turkle (2012). In the context of groups, of course, the question is particularly interesting what the assignment or perceived belonging to a virtual group can mean psychologically.

Let's pick out one aspect of the event and take a closer look at the relationship between virtual groups and presence groups. What influences does the increasing virtuality of group experience have on the "group identity" of the individual?

2.1 Narcissistic Affirmation

First of all, it is undisputed that the possibility of virtual contacts (email, WhatsApp groups, chat groups, etc.) offers a multitude of new options for establishing new contacts, pursuing interests and meeting like-minded people, presenting and articulating oneself, often initially also controlled and selectively, so that the fears of embarrassment and humiliation, which are stronger in presence groups, can have less effect. The phenomenon of "ghosting" is mentioned here as an example, which involves the uncommented termination of a virtual contact, an act that can often cause considerable irritation and anger. Thus, a feared embarrassment is passed on to others without the possibility of clarification, as would be the case in real contact.

The multitude of contact options, whether factual or often only imagined, can trigger a feeling of self-efficacy and power. Someone feels mirrored, accepted, desired, and admired. This narcissistic gratification is an elementary component of virtual contacts on the internet, which can lead to addiction. The sociological background of this development is the strong individualization and the associated loosening of integration into traditional social contexts of post-war societies such as clubs, church communities, etc. This process has been described by Reckwitz (2017) as a development towards a "society of singularities". Turkle (2019) laments the effects of digital empowerment tools on the psyche. Like others (see Lanier 2018; Mozorov 2013), she notes the danger of an increase in isolation, narcissistic personality development, and a manager complex. There is a rampant idea that one must be the controlling instance of life in everything, distilled this is expressed in the non-word "I-AG" for precariously employed pseudo-self-employed.

Lack of Digital Competence

Much suggests that dealing with social media and the internet largely depends on what psychologists recently call "resilience", others, however, "digital competence". It is suspected that digital media pose a great temptation and danger, especially for emotionally unstable people. Isolation and dependence threaten. People who already find it difficult to establish and maintain social contacts will find the promises of social media very tempting. Once again, the disadvantages of innovations in technical terms primarily affect the disadvantaged in society. People with poorer education, with poorer health are at risk of wanting to satisfy their neediness more on the net, as the risk of personal rejection and humiliation seems more manageable there. If someone crosses you, you simply click them away. Less pessimistic about the fear of replacing previous social contact among people with their migration to social networks is Vogelsang (2020). He sees intercorporeality as a prerequisite for the connectedness of people and can only imagine a hybrid mixture of personal and virtual contact forms in the future. "They (the networks) use digital technologies and yet each and every one of them is in continuity with the previous forms of connectedness. Narrativity, localization, physical presence, and conflicts will also shape future forms of connectedness. …" (Vogelsang 2020, p. 212). Thus, the theologian and engineer is much more optimistic than some social science colleagues.

2.2 Calming Instead of Object Constancy

It is obvious how quickly many, perhaps even most people in public spaces, pull out their mobile phone and look at it when they are not immediately engaged in another activity. Free time or moments of embarrassment, waiting times or physical proximity to others enforced by means of transport and routes are usually answered by "diving" into one's virtual bubble. Hardly anyone lets their gaze wander over the passing landscape from a train for several minutes anymore. What is likely happening is that internal moments of tension, emerging affects and feelings of restlessness are being discharged. Looking at the mobile phone becomes a displacement activity, similar to the pecking of caged chickens in the face of the insoluble conflict between flight and fight tendencies, should a fox sneak up. While the mobile phone may also provide desirable auxiliary ego services, such as when a person with a panic disorder is more capable of going into the forest alone than before. The calming fact of always being reachable brings other people (psychoanalytically: objects) closer internally and represses the real situation: One is still possibly kilometers away from any other, real human contact. But psychologically, in the imagination, this is no longer the case. The presence or proximity of another person suggested by the device possibly replaces the internal ability of object constancy, i.e., being able to access the other as a representation within oneself. This could cause this internal psychological performance to not develop as well.

Should the theory be adapted to the changes?
Does this object-relational, analytical thinking therefore need to be expanded? Because the presence of the other as an idea happens quite naturally, on the other hand with reference to and possibly using a mobile phone. Whether this involves different internal psychological processes would need to be investigated. Added to this is the obvious difference to the physical presence of the other. In practice, however, the technical devices seem to have a calming effect, for example in the case of a person suffering from a panic disorder.

So we are dealing with the establishment of a new kind of transitional object in view of the anytime availability of a virtual contact. The other is there and yet not there, but their absence becomes more bearable. If one thinks this through, it is actually over for most people with the absolute retreat, being alone without the immediate possibility of interruption, even in the most remote places on earth. Except in the case where one consciously gives one's mobile phones to someone else for safekeeping before a meditation retreat, a digital abstinence rarely occurs. Research with adolescents shows a steadily increasing usage time (ZEIT-Online 2021; Tagesschau 2023). In treatments and personal conversations, one also hears reports of fierce disputes between parents and children. Withdrawal symptoms sometimes seem to occur, up to panic with a multitude of vegetative symptoms, if one takes the mobile phone away from children or adolescents for only 24 hours. These indications of dependency are partly eminent and pathological according to conventional criteria. However, the question arises whether the criteria for problem analysis are still applicable from the known context or whether the digital change and its effects could be better captured with other concepts. Regarding the agoraphobia patient walking alone in the forest, the technical communication extensions are both enabling and limiting: The latter is that a real internal stability and independence, which could also indicate symptom freedom, can never really be claimed, as the "experimental setup" no longer allows this.

2.3 Attention in Breadth Instead of Depth

Associated with the triumph of digital media and the underlying type of data processing, a new conception of the invisible, the unknown, perhaps also the unconscious seems to be emerging: With the data mining of individuals and the big data approaches of industry, it is suggested that sufficiently large amounts of data will ensure that people can be enlightened about previously unconscious connections and facts as well as that these can then be corrected. The fetish of computing power gives rise to the illusion that the data collected at time X will already reveal their internal connections. Connections that can no longer know anything about the idea of unconscious determinism, of conceptualizations of the human psyche that go deep, and also do not want to, as they also see their goal of successful behavior optimization very close.

The multitude of stimuli and units of information that flood us today, digitally mediated, on the other hand, causes an increasingly broad attention regime. Even the most remote associations of the YouTube algorithms still find their way into our suggestion lists. But these are no longer our own associations, as could be the case in the feedback round of a group, for example.

2.4 Virtual Groups vs. Physical Presence Groups

Many group therapists have been able to try out the most diverse group settings, previously unthinkable for them, during the course of the Covid-19 pandemic. We know what it's like to conduct groups online (these could not be billed to the insurance companies); hybrid groups were also conducted. As a bridge in a difficult time threatening contacts, virtual offerings such as online video conferences were a relief for many. Nevertheless, there is skepticism and a variety of problems (see Münch 2021; Gorvin 2022).

Many people expressed relief after being able to meet again in person for group meetings and group therapies. Many complained about the limitation of experiencing in virtuality (the other person is just a "tile"). Many missed the holistic perception of the physicality of others, including their gestures, facial expressions, eye contact, and smell. Others, especially patients suffering from anxiety or obsessive-compulsive disorders, even as participants in group therapy, tended to withdraw, not show up, or even end their group participation. If the group had not already been experienced as helpful, supportive, and "good enough", then the forced separations and interruptions caused by the pandemic apparently triggered too much abandonment rage, which could then be acted out, as it could not be worked on in the group.

But how do the different experiences in virtuality and presence contact regarding groups interact? Virtual experience and experience of the other in presence do not now take place in two different worlds, but a person must mentally process and integrate these different experiences, often with the same others. In anamneses, there is often still too little asked about the extent of integration into the digital world, although this seems to be a large time of the day for adolescents and young adults. The importance of digital networking and the nature of the internal representation of these contacts and activities alongside the representations of the "real" contacts of the persons concerned should become clear. It could be imagined that frustrations in the real world of contacts are attempted to be compensated by better controllable digital and virtual contacts on the net. Without the complete picture of the inner world of the "others", be they real or virtual contacts, there remains uncertainty and the constant possibility of missing the mark. If I express compassion for the rejection or loneliness of the person concerned, I must take into account whether this person has not simultaneously established himself in grandiose narcissistic defense as a hero in the mastery of a computer game, for which he would rather be admired.

Example

A patient reported that he not only frequently pursued his gaming passion on a parallel monitor during his online working hours, but that he had also occasionally done so during online therapy sessions. He showed himself to be both proud and provocative, but also ashamed, and was even able to reflectively comment on his behavior. ◄

The Consequences of the Covid-19 Pandemic

There are indications that personal contacts will continue to decrease after the pandemic, the more opportunities for digital contact or distraction arise. Teenagers meet in chat rooms, older people no longer go to the theater as often, presence seminars find less approval than the online format, many employees are forced to work from home at least several days a week. All of this suggests that there seems to be an internal overall view in the "accounting" of personal contacts, which should be taken into account in psychotherapies. Many of the previously asked questions about the influence of virtual groups on our understanding of living together and groups, including therapeutic groups, can only be circled associatively here. It should be noted at this point that presence groups seem to be losing and gaining influence at the same time. The contrast of the experiences in the two forms of encounter makes their respective characteristics more recognizable and clarifies advantages and disadvantages. In this respect, one can hope that a process of becoming aware is set in motion, which makes us more aware of our group existence and dependence on groups, the more we threaten to lose the connection to groups through isolation. The processes can therefore be hypostasized as dialectical and, in the sense of the understanding of defense in Analytical Psychology, one can rather ask about the final purpose of the ever new, technical inventions. This is also in line with Giegerich (e.g. 1988), who repeatedly encouraged an integrative view of man's technical affinity.

2.5 Understanding Instead of Defense

Without being able to conclusively answer the questions about the relationship between virtual and real groups at this point: It could prove unfavorable for psychoanalysis if it primarily forms a front against digital innovations. Hardt (2019) saw psychoanalysis in fundamental conflict with the digital revolution, not without reason, but probably with too few visions of a more successful synthesis of human and technology in the future. In this view, humans are defined as too inflexible and unchangeable, it is not taken into account how people have always had to cope with enormous upheavals through epochal breaks in their lives (cf. Bode 2004; Röhl 2022; Utari-Witt and Kogan 2015).

What is important for us at this point is that we always keep in mind in our professional everyday life, but also when further considering the influence of groups on our life path, that digital and virtual contacts should always be considered as a second matrix in the background. Otherwise, one does not do justice to the increasing complexity of events and underestimates once again the influence that groups have on individual development, thereby overlooking an essential piece of psychological reality. It should also be noted that a great deal of research needs to be done in this regard.

2.6 Concepts of Individuation

Our ideas of self-becoming in the face of the impositions and influences of life are manifold. While psychoanalysis has emphasized the development away from unrestricted dependence towards personal autonomy, Jung's analytical psychology speaks of the process of individuation, the "self-becoming", a concept that, despite all openness to transpersonal thoughts (keyword: collective unconscious), was also long understood too one-sidedly introverted, i.e., merely as an inner, personality-forming process. My point here is that we have obviously thought of the individual as too "individual" for long stretches. Because to individuate *against* society is basically an impossible endeavor and not really necessary to live a satisfied life. The idea of a conflict between societal and individual needs is basically an antithesis to what really happens. In the course of the development of an increasingly consumer-oriented lifestyle in our part of the world, the individual has increasingly fallen victim to a neoliberal ideology, more and more areas of life have been subjected to rationality and management-like self-organization demands and necessities (keyword: digitalization; cf. Münch 2021). Society thus already permeates the finest fibers of individual life design and, particularly insidiously, in such a way that the individual usually does not even notice. Many people are even convinced that their consumerist self-realization path is a unique one and exactly as they want it, even though they use the methods and contents of mass media culture. Especially conservative economists and politicians repeatedly present this idea of the self-inventing and always striving for higher (consumption) human being, exaggerated by market logic. This conviction also does not stop at images and ideas of how one's own body (cf. Vedder 2022) and one's own soul could and should be continuously optimized. The societal thus once again merges into the self-definition of the individual and thus becomes harder to decipher.

If one thinks longer about this dynamic, one realizes that belonging to groups also seems to be a motive for the often unconscious behavior of individuals: By joining a collective movement, such as the self-tracking movement, I become part of a larger whole, at least in imagination. This can indeed be experienced as satisfying, at least as long as one deals with the consequences of transmitting the most personal data to other "larger wholes", namely digital corporations. The attempt to overcome isolation is therefore increasingly taking place on the Internet, often in a predominantly constructive way such as in partner search, unfortunately more often also in the form of shitstorms and hate speeches. For the collapsing, meaning-giving, group structures in the real environment, an attempt is made to find a virtual replacement.

2.7 Fallen Out of All Groups: Loneliness

England and Japan already have one: a Ministry of Loneliness. Apparently, governments have recognized that, recently promoted by the pandemic, curfews and compulsory home office, loneliness as a mass phenomenon is increasingly gaining societal and also health policy relevance (cf. Senk 2022). Our societies are breaking down into ever smaller individual units: through digitalization, neglect of public spaces, decline of club ties. More and more people are alone more and more often. In large cities, there is a high proportion of single households, for example in Munich almost 55% of all people live alone. This is certainly also an expression of prosperity, but it also shows how little current small group or family experience people still have. Fittingly, Munich is also a stronghold of psychotherapists, so, seen humorously, at least partial remedy can be provided.

Only the experience of a positively connoted group context can cause a deeper transformation in the worldview. The worldview of being fundamentally separated from others is found in many relationships that I can observe: in the circle of acquaintances, in society, but especially among my patients. In contrast to this is the deeply satisfying experience of a sense of community and coexistence, for which the term "love" (cf. Stuck 2016) would be a possible expression. If one dares to say it like this.

Whoever first asks about the individual, gets the answer from the individual. Those who lack a nourishing group experience, who have never been allowed to experience this, carry no internal concept of it. These patients would hardly ever ask for group experiences on their own. It is like a dark spot on the soul, caused by neglect, indifference, lack of empathy or even abuse in childhood or later. What has actually shaped me, the others who have become part of me, is no longer directly perceptible. Many patients are in great conflict with themselves and are very unfriendly, even judgmental towards themselves, which makes it very difficult for them to get along with themselves and also to have social contacts, as these contacts can easily revive the destructive inner voices in a projective way and cause relationships to fail.

The Distortion of Perception

In psychoanalyses and psychotherapies, psychodynamically oriented helpers try to create a space for new experiences by painstakingly trying to make expectations and transferences in reality more conscious. This names the distortion of experience and makes it perceptible as such. Only when the basic feeling of trustful connection with others is present, do patients slowly venture out of their previous self- and world-image. It can be very enriching and gratifying for psychotherapists when people can say at the end of their group therapeutic time that they now stand at a different point in their inner landscape: having a perspective on themselves that has been made possible through the reflection, the conscious and above all unconscious interaction with the other group participants. The own psychological position is then enriched and changed by the contact with the internalized group experience. This proves the "inner groupality" (Kaes 2009) of every human being not only as an enrichment, but even as a prerequisite of his individuality.

Expanding our View of Groups

Dalal (1998) ultimately does not call for a reversal of our perspective on the individual and his development, but for an expansion of our view. This is what I would like to encourage with this book. What if we try to see the human being and his psyche first from the perspective of the group and the fact of the human being's embeddedness in his groups? Anyone who approaches the individual from this side would be able to identify even more conditioning factors than the often only slightly reconstructable historical-biographical experiences. This could protect against false illusions and some disappointments, also the patients from their often distorted assessments of reality due to their high neediness. The fact that the trusting relationship with their therapist alone can initiate a change is a necessary but not sufficient condition for therapeutic success. This also means: Without an idealizing transference to the group therapists, participation in a group is difficult. The obstacles on the way towards recovery are relatively often in the environmental factors to which people are exposed parallel to therapy. A group can help correct these assumptions much faster, as the regressive sliding is caught by several others. Someone who has too great illusions about fulfillment in a partnership, often also has these expectations in the idealized one-to-one relationship with the therapist. Here, the dyadic becomes a fetish, the togetherness a promise of salvation, which no imperfect human being in the world is capable of fulfilling.

Groups Facilitate Change Processes
Those who intend to change on their own often quickly encounter limits, namely the lack of willingness to change on the part of others, including the structures in familial or work-related groups. Group therapies themselves, however, are an alternative structure to these disease-causing environments. Understanding and considering this would be a gain. Only rarely can a form of positive "contagion" be observed in the environment of patients due to the insights and psychological growth processes achieved in the therapy of the respective patients. Much more often, entire teams show a tendency to resist individuals who want to change. Especially from this point of view, the consideration of the groups in which someone is involved is of high relevance. This is not to say that such aspects are not often touched upon in individual treatments. In my opinion, however, group influences are often still not sufficiently taken into account in their significance for the psychological structure of the individual. Rather, people often still think in terms of one-sided or mutual influence, interaction or opposition of individual human groups. The approach represented here goes beyond that. It is a radical application of what Elias (cited according to Dalal 1998) has already described as the "social unconscious" and also of what C. G. Jung tried to describe as the dissociability of the psyche and the "objective psyche". It is about thinking the indivisibility of the seemingly separate unit individual-group. In each case, it is not about hypostasizing a resting center of the experiencer and thus of the subject "subjected" to the environment, but about a movable, never stable image of the dynamics of becoming (cf. Voigt 2019) and of co-constructivity as a design principle of psychological development (cf. Orange 2015; Lesmeister 2009), to create, hold and thus be able to better meet the shared psychological reality.

How diversely one can experience being connected and bonded with other people, with ideas and values, with nature, even as a person living alone, is impressively reported by Daniel Schreiber in his essay *Alone* (2022).

2.8 Affiliation and the Archetypal Heritage

The success of human history so far is due to a history of cooperation among groups of people. In his book *Humankind: A Hopeful History*, Bregman (2019) describes through many examples that the history of humanity should not be understood merely as an endless succession of wars, plagues, and disasters, but as a result of the ultimately dominant ability for cooperation and creative transformation. It is assumed that the experiences of tens of thousands of years of human coexistence can be found in the human genome. We actually expect the other! We deeply believe that we do not have to remain alone and that we can go through life in connection. This is also indicated by psychoanalytical and sociological studies. Braten (2011) speaks of the "virtual other" who exists as an expectable idea in us even before we encounter the real other as an infant. This primary experience, deeply rooted in our history, if disappointed, can make us doubt ourselves, the other, and the world, so that mental illness can arise. Groups are the context in which this can be answered in the most natural way through an offer in the here and now. They also fundamentally question the assumption that one can accomplish anything entirely alone without others. And rightly so. Mental health can only be achieved in encounters with other people. If this contact is missing too much, one feels fallen out of the community of the living, of life, and of time.

The Ego-Self Axis

Neumann (cf. Löwe 2014) spoke of the relationship between our ego, the everyday consciousness, and the much more comprehensive self as the source of our powers and also our destiny. This inner connection can also be discovered and strengthened in groups. In groups, these forces can be personally experienced. There is a connection between the experience of direct personal exchange about experiences and feelings and the strengthening of the relationship to the inner world. The others are always simultaneously a medium for exploring one's own, perhaps hitherto only projected, and at the same time the others, whose otherness wants to be recognized by me. Self-recognition, self-knowledge can only succeed if I am able to recognize the other, also as a foreigner. Recognition means real listening, the deep experience that there is someone outside of me who has something important to tell me about myself. This process happens in a group for all participants at the same time and naturally at different speeds and sustainably due to different conditions. Someone who is too much caught by his fear of his own unpleasant sides, in other words, someone who rejects a lot, can also hardly achieve an opening for the views of others, as this activates fear. The other becomes the enemy, the attacker, against whom one thinks one has to defend oneself, instead of one's own inner fought.

Group experience can help to gradually change and, with the consideration of others, who also experience this process of transformation, achieve more self-opening, self-knowledge, and less projection. Life becomes more manageable and easier when others no longer have to be seen as the source of my suffering, but when someone finds instances within themselves that devalue, but also express self-acceptance and appreciation. Since this is not an easy and pleasant process, the help of the presence of others as witnesses, as helpers and "others" in the sense of a counterpart that also confronts and "imposes" itself, is extremely important and can lead to profound, even structural mental changes. Above all, however, the others "carry" one towards a gradually more comprehensive recognition of one's own person, including one's own weaknesses.

References

Altmeyer, M, Kächele, H (2006) Die vernetzte Seele. Klett-Cotta, Stuttgart

Bode, S (2004) Die vergessene Generation. Klett-Cotta, Stuttgart

Braten, S (2011) Intersubjektive Partizipation: Bewegungen des virtuellen Anderen bei Säuglingen und Erwachsenen. Psyche 9/10: 832-861

Bregman, R (2019) Im Grunde gut. Rowohlt, Hamburg

Elias, N (1994) The Civilizing Process. Blackwell, Oxford

Giegerich, W (1988) Die Atombombe als seelische Wirklichkeit. Schweizer Spiegel Verlag, Zürich
Gorvin, G (2022) Online-Video-Gruppen—Eindrücke und Reflexionen während der Covid-19-Pandemie. Gruppenpsychother. Gruppendynamik 58: 27–40. Vandenhoeck & Ruprecht, Göttingen
Hardt, J (2019) Psychoanalyse im Widerstreit mit der digitalen Welt. In: Psyche 73,9: 826–851
Kaes, R (2009) Innere Gruppen und psychische Gruppalität: Entstehung und Hintergründe eines Konzepts. Psyche 63C(3): 281-305
Lanier, J (2018) Anbruch einer neuen Zeit. Hoffmann und Campe, Hamburg
Lesmeister, R (2009) Selbst und Individuation. Brandes & Apsel Verlag, Frankfurt/M
Löwe, A (2014) Auf Seiten der inneren Stimme. Karl-Alber-Verlag, Baden-Baden
Mozorov, E (2013) To save everything click here. Penguin, London
Münch, V (2021) Angriffe auf die Seele. Brandes & Apsel Verlag, Frankfurt/M
Orange, D (2015) Intersubjektivität in der Psychoanalyse. Brandes & Apsel Verlag, Frankfurt/M
Reckwitz, A (2017) Die Gesellschaft der Singularitäten. Suhrkamp, Berlin
Röhl, A (2022) Das Elend der Verschickungskinder. Psychosozial-Verlag, Gießen
Schreiber, D (2022) Allein. Suhrkamp, Berlin
Senk, J (2022) Braucht Deutschland ein Einsamkeitsministerium? https://www.domradio.de/artikel/braucht-deutschland-ein-einsamkeitsministerium, 15.6.2022, (Stand: 18.12.2022)
Stuck, U (2016). Plädoyer für den Gruppengedanken in der Analytischen Psychologie. Selbst, Ich und Wir. Brandes und Apsel Verlag, Frankfurt/M
Türcke, C (2012) Hyperaktiv. Beck'sche Reihe, München
Turkle, S (2012) Verloren unter 100 Freunden. Riemann, München
Turkle, S (2019) Empathie-Maschinen. Psyche 73,9: 726–743. Klett-Cotta, Stuttgart
Utari-Witt, H., Kogan I (Hrsg) (2015) Unterwegs in der Fremde. Psychosozial-Verlag, Gießen
Vedder, B (2022) Solidarische Körper. Büchner-Verlag, Marburg
Vogelsang, F (2020) Soziale Verbundenheit. Verlag Karl Alber, München
Voigt B (2019) Vom Werden. Beatrice Voigt Edition, München

The First Groups: Prenatal Development, Birth, Early Childhood, Latency Period

3

Abstract

Here begins our journey through the course of life. We aim to understand how deeply and sustainably we are integrated into group contexts during our lifelong development, and how dependent we are on them, and we will see how little this has been considered in many treatment settings that are designed solely for individual therapy. Whenever we use the terms kindergarten, class, team, work group, band, shared apartment, relatives, we are essentially talking about group contexts. However, our imprinting begins even before we appear in the world.

To sharpen awareness of what Foulkes or Elias mean by the "social unconscious," it should be clarified that all of our psychic lives are already shaped long before our birth. As we know from daily work with patients, not only the conflicts and neurotic relationship structures prevalent in a person or a family are relevant to understanding symptoms. Every utterance, every life path also makes the image of a patient's origin clearer. The way they dress, how they speak, and even how they move, says a lot. Often it is the social background, ultimately the intellectual and cultural imprint of the parental home, that has a decisive influence on a person's self-understanding and worldview. A patient who comes from poor circumstances, patients who could not grow up with their biological parents, who have been adopted, who have a history of being in a home or who have grown up with foster parents, have a completely different worldview and different value standards than people from wealthy, at least outwardly successful families. Hobbies, leisure activities, and interests often differ significantly. It is still noticeable that our society consists of different social backgrounds, formerly called classes, which often have little contact with each other. When these differently shaped people meet in

V. Münch, *Group Experience as a Resource*,
https://doi.org/10.1007/978-3-662-70864-4_3

group psychotherapy, this can lead to communication problems, alienation, even conflicts. But it can also lead to mutual enrichment, to the expansion of personal horizons. In this respect, group therapies also have a socially balancing function (cf. Geyer 2023).

Transgenerational Trauma Transmission

Before a person comes into the world, their parents already have a history in this world. This was largely shaped by their own parents. This continues through the generations backwards. If the parents were born in the now past century, many of the grandparents and great-grandparents experienced traumatic events in connection with war, flight, or displacement. All of this significantly influences the atmosphere in a family. If severe experiences have to be coped with, repression often prevails, which leads to the unconscious transmission of traumas, referred to as transgenerational transmission of traumas. All of this happens unconsciously and without having to be verbally thematized. It is precisely the silence that leads to children being born into a world that is emotionally incomprehensible and full of secrets for them. Bode (2004) and Lorenz (2003) have made this clear to a broad section of the population in moving books in Germany. The large group experiences and group experiences of participants of the 2nd World War are therefore also present in the psyche of the descendants and influence their experiences and behavior in groups.

When taking a medical history and the associated intensive questioning of patients, it is now at least standard in analytical procedures that the life stories of grandparents and of course parents are also extensively recorded. But this always also asks into which groups someone was integrated, with which group-organizing ideologies (cf. Dalal 1998) someone might be identified and what role someone has played in social groups of various kinds or whether someone has led a rather withdrawn life. It seems strange from today's perspective to imagine that psychotherapy has long followed the assumption of the mind as a monad. C. G. Jung had already tried to correct this view. Certainly, the fact that this ideology was very entrenched in society plays a role, as the impression arose at least in the second half of the 20th century that human autonomy development could achieve considerable successes, also with regard to technology and economy. In view of mass phenomena and thus also groups, people were understandably very negative against the background of Nazism and Stalinism.

Critical: The Large Group as a Mass Phenomenon

The realization that psychological life could always be thought of as group-based before any individuation, and thus ultimately always represents a selected, albeit remarkable, section of a larger whole, has only recently become more apparent to us. More on the question of why we need a collective, communal, group-based thinking to better cope with our problems on a societal and subsequently also on an individual level, is said in the second part of the book. Especially after the horrific aberrations of the Nazi era and its mass phenomena, its regression and its excesses of violence, it was all too plausible that only the ethically responsible, individual human being (Neumann 1993) appeared as the standard for a successful future. The construction of a new world from the ruins was ultimately only possible together, also with the help of understandable and necessary collective repression (cf. Mitscherlich and Mitscherlich-Nielsen 1985). The responsibility of individuals for success or failure was strongly emphasized. *Now* everyone should be able to forge their own fortune, based on performance and ambition. Thus, in the early Federal Republic of Germany, there were a number of ideals that were difficult to criticize, whose adherence soon led to modest prosperity and the experience that one's own efforts could contribute to constructive and generally appreciated things. The collective large group experiences and societal atmospheres that accumulated in individuals led to hope, optimism, and readiness to act. One of these readiness to act is the desire to have children. Although this is experienced as one's own wish, it also serves the continuation of society, which usually signals an interest in sufficient offspring and provides the conditions for it.

No matter what time parents live in, they are always embedded in the traumas, dreams, and fears of previous generations, and this in a complicated, nested, and multi-layered way. The ideal that some parents develop, namely to make as few "mistakes" as possible and not to pass on any unresolved conflicts and issues of their parents and other ancestors, is unfulfillable: Life itself seems to be an "event" that offers only gradual and usually incomplete processing of past experiences and also imposes on descendants their share in coping with long-past human catastrophes. Part of this can be worked through in psychotherapies.

Helpful Understanding of Large Group Dynamics

The German-British consultant and group analyst Gerhard Wilke (2017) has humorously and intricately illustrated how the traumas of previous generations indirectly and intricately influence the psychological life of people living today, especially in group contexts (see Chap. 16). His analyses of the aftereffects of the past in the group dynamics of even experienced clinicians and therapists point out how little self-evident the reflection of these levels of our behavior and experience is and how necessary a greater awareness is to counteract misdevelopments, conflicts, and disputes. Especially in times of diverse tendencies towards division, we need such integrative tools as guided large group events (see Chap. 16). On the topic of the consequences of climate change, we are currently experiencing this in a drastic and overly clear way. Rarely has it been so collectively conscious and at least acknowledged on the attitude side that we bear a responsibility for the future of our children and are very inadequately fulfilling it. Some younger people today say that they could no longer justify having children. This is thought-provoking and a sign that a completely new way of thinking is required.

The future mother and father are thus embedded in their groups: in their family of origin, in circles of friends, in work groups, in interest-led groups in their free time, in the atmospheres of society. This may seem banal, but it is crucial if one is willing to think of human development as embedded in a group event. Because this is not about the factual encounter of these people with others on the outside, but about the structure of their psyche, which is a group one, characterized by diversity. The ideas of belonging, connection, loyalty, and exchange constitute the individual psyche. Even the ideas about the unborn child, which at this point only exists in the imagination, are influenced by this. Today we know a lot about the influences of the prenatal period, the mother's environment, the early development of the sense of hearing in particular, and we see the prenatal, perinatal, and postnatal world not as completely separate, but as a process for the experience of the baby and also the parents. Certainly, birth has the most important meaning here, as it is a dangerous and symbolically charged threshold situation.

3.1 Replacement Children

An important anamnestic question concerns so-called replacement children: If the mother has had a miscarriage, an abortion, or in some other way lost a child due to an accident or illness before the birth of the patient, this often has a detrimental effect on the next-born child. This child is confronted with the mother's (loss-) fears and her partly unresolved grief, or in the case of unprocessed loss, with the mother's depressive symptoms. This causes, especially when it hits the child particularly early and thus particularly sustainably and at the same time unconsciously, that in adulthood sometimes difficult to describe and diffuse depressive states can develop. In this case, the old structure of the family group has an unconscious, destructive influence on the development of the person concerned. This often never discussed, but all the more effective unconscious influence of the family group and its unconscious on the mental development of the then newly born, is a too often overlooked characteristic of the group influence on mental development. I know numerous patients who find it extremely difficult to find or conquer their place in life due to this dynamic. It is as if they have another task to fulfill, which naturally is not within their power. Thus, they sacrifice their own mental life to make the mother's real loss of a child's life bearable.

Changes in the Zeitgeist

Another dimension naturally influences our becoming and is often overlooked: time. Although it is possible, but perhaps also cheap, if we investigate and sense the causes of neurotic symptoms 50 years after a childhood. From today's perspective, many aspects of the mentality of the time, the way people interacted with each other, the methods of education are questionable. But the prevailing zeitgeist ensured that things that we today naturally view critically could not be reflected on at the time. There is a danger of applying today's standards to what has already happened when looking back at the past, thereby overlooking essential characteristics of this past, also by too quickly evaluating it as merely harmful. Being embedded in the other, then social world, felt very different for those affected than applying today's standards suggests. What I am talking about are the necessities of early repression due to the much greater proximity of trauma and the horror of war. Oskar Roehler describes this very forcefully in his novel *The Lack* (2020) and also in his films. The behavior and moods of their parents were only puzzling for many children at the time because the parents themselves were also strangers to themselves. The collective awareness of such processes has since grown significantly, as has the understanding that we always also examine and try to influence the effects of such earlier collective large group ideologies in psychotherapies taking place today.

3.2 The Birth

The birth itself is a process that can only be managed well if the parents, and especially the mother, feel supported by a group of helping people. The function of the midwife goes far beyond advisory and technical explanations. She is a companion on a special section of the life path. The support of the partner, but also of one's own mother, becomes very significant especially at the birth of the first child. In indigenous cultures, it is the women who take the birthing woman into their midst, calm her, sing, give her the feeling that she is held and that the process of birth, as everyday as it appears, also always carries a numinous and unfathomable side within it. In other words: the others connect with the layers of collective knowledge, the collective unconscious, as C. G. Jung called it. When personal experience is not enough to bear fears and uncertainty, then the knowledge and presence of others can contribute to not feeling left alone, on the contrary, perhaps even to feel connected in a strengthening way with all women, including those of one's own ancestral line, who have experienced similar things.

Internal Representations of Groups

I have already spoken about the multitude of real people and their inner psychic representations in the mother, as they already exist before the birth, indeed before the conception of a new human being. Their inner images form a psychic group, which, despite all possible polyphony, represents an enrichment for the experience. The individual participants of these "groups" do not need to know each other in reality, nor do they need to have ever met. What is important is only the psychological significance that the prospective mother assigns to the inner images of these people. She connects these images with emotional associations. Thus, one could suspect everything from reassurance to disquiet, depending on the qualities these internalized relationships have. If a person is less suitable to function as a supporter, there are (hopefully) inner others who help to compensate for the lack and who calm, give courage and hope as helpful inner objects. The group identity of the parents thus directly and indirectly affects the new life.

3.3 Early Childhood

Plato spoke of the "Daimon", which is assigned to all of us on our life's journey, and Hillman (2002) elaborated on this within his considerations of archetypal psychology. This figure is thought of as a life companion, a guardian of the right, inner path. Sloterdijk (1998) links the origin of this idea with the fact that the first counterpart is not a human, psychoanalytically speaking not a whole object, but rather a "non-object": He identifies the placenta as a nourishing, conceivable, yet unconscious Other, a counterpart from which we would also be abruptly separated, but this usually does not lead to a kind of nostalgic longing. This would, however, be displaced onto many later objects and then be all the more noticeable. Many of our sufferings, such as our search for the perfect partner, can be understood as the never-ending search for this lost first counterpart and also the non-understanding and non-acceptance of the necessary failure of this search in psychotherapies, according to Sloterdijk in his associations.

Children Need Group Experiences

Parents pave the way for their child into social groups at an early stage. If they themselves live in isolation, whether geographically or emotionally distant from other people, then children in their preschool years have few contacts with other children. Only children are even more disadvantaged in this situation.

Example

I remember some patients who lived in such small towns that there were no other children available for arranging playdates. At the same time, relatives of the family lived as neighbors on site. If there were tensions and disputes between the parents and their parents or other relatives, the children felt this and could do little to counteract this situation. If there are few opportunities to exchange with others, fear, insecurity, and tension remain in the psychological system and quickly lead to temporary solutions and symptoms. Often, there is an early retreat into a fantasy world. The grandiose fantasies contained in it try to compensate for the experienced powerlessness, the shame, and the helplessness. These processing takes place completely unconsciously for the child in question and are therefore often invisible to the parents. The lack of contact with other children in the earliest and early years can thus be formative for later difficulties in making contact with others, as concrete, interactive experiences with real others are lacking. ◄

First Group Experiences Within and Outside the Family

From an early age, when toddlers first come into contact with each other, whether through their parents' contacts or through childcare such as daycare centers or similar, children show a natural interest in each other. If this is sufficiently promoted and moderated (by settling disputes, for example), important early experiences are internalized and the detachment from the parents can gradually begin through these experiences with others, with third parties. The increasing independence from parents in childhood and adolescence is primarily reassured by the fact that someone is capable of successfully making contacts with people who are not part of the family and who bring something new, different, and complementary into the psychological world. Talents and interests often develop along the ideas and influences of friends and acquaintances, which can also be caregivers or teachers. Since parents can never share all of the interests and passions of their own offspring, this is an evolutionarily sensible development. However, there is also the risk of maldevelopment from an early stage. There are always children who find it harder to separate from their parents, usually still mainly from the mother, for example when it comes to transitioning to kindergarten. Children who develop fear and psychosomatic complaints such as stomach ache, children who cry a lot, depend on an appropriate handling of these reactions. If the emotions are ignored, it is learned that they are unwanted and therefore to be repressed. Psychosomatic defense formations can begin to form or even a "false self" (cf. Winnicott 1974). If a child's fears are perceived as excessively worrying, this fear can have an intensifying effect on the symptoms, creating a vicious circle in which the child above all does not learn enough: to calm itself. Hyperactive, dramatizing behavior, psychosomatic complaints, and a difficult social role both in the context of contact between parents and caregivers, such as in the "ADHD syndrome", but especially also among peers, can quickly solidify. The inner loneliness, the misunderstanding of the children only becomes greater as a result.

Example

A 43-year-old patient reports about his 12-year-old son who withdraws a lot in his free time. He himself was also a loner at this age, read a lot, and did crafts. With his son, this seems to be repeating itself with computer games. However, we notice that he himself has remained somewhat of a loner to this day, does not have a large circle of friends, and rarely receives or pays visits. So, the son is copying everything from his father at the behavioral level. Appeals for him to make arrangements fall on deaf ears, and little changes. Together, we look for the reasons behind his own isolation. ◀

In this context, it is also important not to overlook the historical developments. For example, 50, 40 years ago in West Germany, it was not as common as it is today to have children cared for in daycare centers and nurseries in order to be able to work. This sometimes controversially discussed fact, however, leads early in the children's lives to them being able to learn how to navigate in group contexts. Nevertheless, it is of course important to pay attention to the suitability for the child. It is quickly possible to overwhelm a child and create the impression that as a child one only has a secondary importance in the parents' lives.

3.3.1 Siblings

One could say that siblings form the first group of equals, so to speak, of people on an equal footing. In any case, siblings can be perceived as the first allies against the parents, an important triangulating process. But usually it is more complicated. While siblings always deal with the same two parents, except in the more complicated case of step-parents and half-siblings, each child reacts differently to the people they encounter. In some families, the already existing siblings represent the first contact with those others who otherwise have to be sought outside the family: other children. Without really understanding what is happening to you, you are fixed in your sibling position, have older siblings who are envied on the one hand, but to whom responsibility for the younger sibling may already have been assigned on the other hand. Then there are the younger siblings, who often develop jealousy because they can steal your attention. Those who grow up without siblings may wonder why they are left so alone, why parental love was not capable of more. Family and siblings cannot be chosen. They are the group that forms due to blood relationship. Every other, every later group always consists of elective affinities. The relationships among siblings are often unconsciously shaped by their parents' sibling relationships, much is imitated, what cannot be imitated is rarely dared, much seems to repeat itself. The later view of one's own siblings in psychotherapy can also help to better understand one's own role within the family structure. With which attributions did one identify early on: the oddball, the ambitious one, the neglected middle child that no one cares about? Children always fight for both closeness and contact as well as recognition for their own talents, characteristics and interests. If the prevailing family legend tends to lump everyone together, offspring with unusual characteristics quickly feel like unwanted outsiders. All of this becomes "live" experience and negotiable again in a therapeutic group.

The Sibling Group
Siblings, especially when they form a small group, can also provide a lot of balance and comfort for the sometimes inevitable injustices they experience through their parents. Especially in precarious families, siblings quickly take on the role of substitute parents, they become parentified, identify with the role of the "better" adult, try to be someone for their sister or brother that they themselves painfully miss. This often triggers problematic developments, even if the unconscious defense strategy initially promises to be helpful. Due to their differences, also due to the order of the sibling series and their different ages, children enter into a different interaction with their parents. They each take on a different role in the family structure, which often has to do with unfulfilled and little integrated parts of their parents. The always restless and conspicuous youngest son, for example, expresses that there are a lot of unspoken conflicts behind the facade of the desired harmonious and adapted mood. The dreamy and rather musically gifted child occupies the place of the "romantic" perhaps also because it is still unoccupied within the family, because there is an unconscious attempt to establish a balance in the family system in order to stabilize it.

3.3.2 Early Trauma and Defense

In many therapies, we witness how patients have adapted very early to the unspoken conditions of their early environment. The psychological legacy of the parents plays a special role here. Unprocessed own traumas, deficits, desires, fears, and other feelings are perceptible to the very small child, albeit not consciously. All the more, however, the parents' defense systems are introjected and thus become part of one's own, unconscious personality. If one realizes that for a child there can be no conceivable other environment, no other first other, then one can tune into the extent of this dependency. What is added from the perspective of Analytical Psychology already in the infant, however, is the archetypal expectation of a sufficiently good parent.

Archaic and Radical Defense Processes

If the expectable and also necessary environment of an accepting, carrying, and holding maternal or paternal environment is not found, archaic defense processes quickly start in the child. To protect its own inner self, its own vitality, the child resorts to a series of "tricks" that we count among the early defense mechanisms, e.g., splitting, projection, and also affect isolation, a very common defense process in cumulative attachment and relationship traumas. To protect itself from further injury, the child can develop an early "false self", which is much more deeply anchored than, for example, the personality part that Jungian psychologists call "persona", as it serves to adapt to different social contexts in adulthood.

A special group of patients are, according to my observation and that of others, people who spent their childhood in the former GDR. Many of them have been in nurseries, sometimes in so-called weekly nurseries, have suffered early frustrations and separations that have remained very unconscious. Often these patients show feelings of resentment and anger that seem incomprehensible to them. Very quickly they feel at the mercy and as victims, can trust very little that open communication and calm handling of conflicts could help them progress.

The Self-Care System

Kalsched (1996) has described in great detail how an inner system develops that is supposed to help compensate for the disappointing real experience. He speaks of the "self-care system", which helps to build an inner fantasy world as a compensation for the frustrating reality, thus maintaining hope by shielding the innermost vital core of the personality from further contact with the outside world as a result of the trauma. This fits well with Jung's basic assumption of the final orientation of all psychic events. To protect the soul from further damage, some outwardly strange and neurotic views and behaviors serve to protect the (still) unaffected vital parts of the person until a sufficiently trustworthy environment can support their development. This can be the moment when one enters into a beneficial relationship, such as psychotherapy.

If the primary family has deeply imprinted itself as the first fateful group experience into the psychic development, it can later in life be very difficult to experience groups as a context in which one can assert oneself and even unfold. This is where the great fear of many patients of groups comes from. This fear is understandable, as one fears not having any internal points of reference to be able to move successfully in a group. If this were not to succeed, it would end in a retraumatizing experience. Here one can only very carefully accept these fears, name them and make them understandable, then they generally also reduce.

3.3.3 Child Dispatch Homes

In the medical histories of people aged around 50 and over, it should also be ascertained whether they were "sent" to children's convalescent homes, which was more common in the past of Western Germany. Röhl (2022), but also Lorenz (2021) have launched initiatives in recent years with great commitment, with the help of which former "dispatch children" can exchange experiences, and they have also published several books on the topic. With justifications still influenced by the Nazi terminology of toughening up and adaptation, children were brought into houses for 6 long weeks, often under the strict regime of doctors and "aunts" (as the child carers, often without proper training, were called by the children). There, communal rooms had to be occupied, even small children had to undertake forced marches of several hours (without food!). Meals that were rejected, sometimes even their own vomit, had to be forcibly consumed. Phone calls did not take place, letters took several days, parents' gifts were distributed to all children. The reports are similar, although there are several hundred different homes. Over 30 years between the 1950s and 1980s, probably around 10 million children were "dispatched". The children exposed to these conditions were socialized differently, so the weaker ones were automatically suppressed and bullied by the stronger ones. So it was anything but a pleasure for children who may already have been suffering from their family circumstances and who had therefore developed psychosomatic symptoms, but rather a further traumatization. There are patients who told me that after 6 weeks in such a home they no longer recognized their parents.

Example

A patient in his 50s reported that he had been sent to a home run by nuns twice for 6 weeks each. The pediatricians had thought that such a stay could strengthen his constitution, sensitivities and allergies as well as his poor nutritional status and also improve his anxiety in contact with other children (!). On site, however, he found no connection, he comforted himself on the long hikes with the sensations associated with experiencing nature: the smell of resin, the taste of blueberries still remind him of this time today. Particularly bad was that he almost choked on his own vomit one night, he had shamefully approached one of the caregivers. After the second of these stays, he was bullied at school by an older, "fat" classmate who had also been on the stay. The bullying, which he could not talk about with anyone at the time, consisted of him being ambushed in every big break and put in a headlock for several minutes without anyone intervening. The problem only disappeared when the boy was transferred in the normal rotation. In his later school life and beyond, he had great fears of others, especially physically active and stronger boys, always felt weak, but for example developed the fantasy of fighting lions victoriously as "Tarzan". In his group therapy, his narcissistic grandiose ideas were initially clearly visible, which is why it was only very slowly possible for him to establish contacts with others. This was initially successful mainly with similarly structured co-patients. Gradually more security was established, less unconscious aggression had to be projected onto the group. The group was perceived as less persecuting, first relationship initiations and bonds crystallized out, which gave and carried security. ◀

Forcing children into groups too early can also promote very unpleasant developments. Much depends on the nature of the primary group, i.e. the family of origin. If this provides enough security and safety, a child can also find the courage to deal with new groups that expand the original group experience. Otherwise, fears prevent new experiences from being made and integrated. It is important that children regularly return to their own family after a period of care by non-family members. The change between different group contexts is very stimulating and instructive. In this way, the often unspoken basic assumptions about human behavior and experience, which underlie many behaviors, can be sensed. This can help to better understand the original group of origin and to gradually relativize the experiences made there. This can help support the process of detachment from the primary group.

3.3.4 The Parental Fallacy following Hillman

Everything said here about the influence of parents on the development of their children does not mean that they alone are to blame for the occurrence of psychological damage in their children. As a rule, it is not individual traumas and events, but rather atmospheres and attitudes that are "inhaled" over decades that lead to the formation of negative introjects. Jung's student Hillman referred to this in *Character and Destiny* (2002) as the "parental fallacy". He emphasizes the role of disposition, talent, and archetypal equipment of the individual. He considers it too short-sighted to view a person as a tabula rasa, who is at the mercy of his external world from birth and is shaped by it.

Bärfuss (2022) also opposes an one-sided overemphasis of parental influence in an autobiographically influenced publication for other reasons. The entire view of individuals in our society would be directed towards origin and ancestors. He also sees social reasons in this, such as the defense against unwanted migration into higher social classes. People should remember their roots also for the reason not to "betray" their own social group, not to abandon it. In this respect, the codes within such social groups would be passed on from generation to generation. In this respect, one can once again see how much our ideas of socialization are shaped by whether we agree with the prevailing form of society. A more group-oriented view of the individual's becoming also emphasizes the great influence of injustices and disadvantages of entire social groups and therefore represents a political issue.

Why, as mentioned, group therapy also has a stronger political implication will be discussed in more detail elsewhere (see Chap. 16, 17).

3.3.5 Aggressive Behavior in Children

From an early age, some children stand out due to aggressive behavior. They quickly become scapegoats in groups, such as in daycare, kindergarten, or school, the dynamics intensify and quickly divide the environment. With their conspicuous behavior, such children draw attention to their inner tensions. Since adapted, quiet behavior is generally desired in groups in daycare and kindergarten, and especially in school, this often leads to major problems. Behavior that is directed against the group can also be referred to as "anti-group behavior" with Nitsun (2014). This makes the individual a symptom carrier of an unconscious readiness for aggression in groups. According to Nitsun, these aggressive to destructive tendencies are present in every group, but they do not become equally virulent everywhere. If the dynamics are not recognized, scapegoats are quickly established. Certain children express aggression for others. The result: Their own aggression remains unconscious. If a conversation about it is started, there is also the chance that other, "quiet" children in their group learn to deal with their anger and aggression more consciously and constructively. This can also sharpen self-perception.

3.3.6 Triangulating Groups

The distancing from the parental home, which as a detachment process already goes hand in hand with every triangulating contact within, but then especially outside the family throughout childhood and adolescence, is driven and promoted by an appropriate selection of contacts with others and their groups. Triangulation, dealing with a triadic constellation, is an elementary developmental step (Grieser 2015). Groups always offer a multitude of constellations, because every contact with another group member puts the others in a different position. Then there is the best friend, the best girlfriend, and the others. These could react jealously or envy the pair of friends, they could feel excluded. The same could happen if a group unites against two children and they join forces. Groups always cause fear and this fear is usually met in such a way that one looks at what and who seems more familiar in the still unfamiliar environment. Thus, we find people who seem similar to us more sympathetic and we are more likely to befriend them. Thus, friendships in the form of subgroups within the larger group form quite quickly in a large group, such as in kindergarten. These smaller units provide security because they are more manageable. More frequent contact with individuals creates an increasing atmosphere of familiarity and thus also strengthens the ego, so that one does not feel too uncomfortable even in unfamiliar situations in which the closest friends are not present. Thus, tolerance for unpleasant feelings is strengthened.

Holding Environment
From Winnicott's *Theory of the Parent-Child Relationship* (1960), it can also be inferred that a group can be seen as a variant of the "environmental mother", that necessary "holding environment" for appropriate development, which facilitates the patients' confrontation with the object-mother. What does this mean for the situation in kindergarten? The large group of children led by the leaders, and even the institution "kindergarten" itself, create an atmosphere of care and moderate incentives (others, games, explorations on excursions) in the best case scenario. This could also be referred to as a "group skin" that is capable of protecting against internal and external threats. Against this background, subgroups and dyadic relationships now form. The original psychological space with the mother (and the family) at home is essentially expanded or doubled. This gives a child more independence from the primary family and learns to perceive itself in other aspects and also to position itself against the wishes of the mother or father and to communicate this. The inner security that can result from anchoring in the new group environment is itself the most important triangulation in this time of first encounters with others in the first non-family groups.

Attachment Styles According to Bowlby
But in order to be able to benefit from a group context in this way, even the smaller child needs a sufficiently secure attachment to the primary caregivers. If it is feared that relationships with others could destroy the bond by moving too far away from them, the necessary freedom for exploratory behavior is not given. Insecure-ambivalent and insecure-avoidant attached children are now at a disadvantage, of course especially those with a disorganized attachment style (cf. Grossmann and Grossmann 2015). They can only inadequately use the new relationship offers for their emancipative development: they remain shy, introverted and have only a few contacts. For people with already serious childhood traumas, the extreme vulnerability resulting from this can quickly lead to retraumatizing experiences. Others sense this and withdraw more quickly. A vicious circle is created that cements inner loneliness.

Conversely, positive relationship experiences in the parental home with a secure attachment can be used to allow new experiences with others and thus new attachments. A group is experienced internally like an object. Depending on previous experiences with the objects (inner images of the people) of the primary family, groups are either sought or avoided, encountered with fear or curiosity, group experiences are rather associated with pleasure or displeasure. These imprints happen very early. In the house where my practice is, there is a kindergarten on the ground floor, and when I look into the garden in the morning, about 25 3- and 4-year-olds are running around. It is impressive how differently the children behave socially. Some romp in community with others, others stand a little apart or seem to be waiting longingly for their parents at the fence. It seems that dealing with others and the feeling of belonging to a group already arises early and is very behavior-guiding.

The Neglect of Group Influence

In addition to Hillman's emphasis on the innate, the archetypal, the talents brought along, we can list the social group and its influence, which significantly influences the development of individual people. This is particularly visible in another aspect of societal-family life, which has been solidifying for decades. I am talking about the dominance of the nuclear family, which often gets into spirals of overburdening. If there are few siblings or relatives such as grandparents or uncles and aunts present, there are fewer opportunities to experience other perspectives, to find a balance for perhaps one-sided reactions or injustices on the part of the parents. Like in a greenhouse, psychosocial conflicts and their internal effects on structural development against this background intensify much faster. In treatments it becomes clear: Many patients find a balance for childhood frustrations through their grandparents. The memories of these are often internalized as positive introjects. If the experiences with both parents were very stressful and insufficient, this is often important for therapy. Because in this way a patient is able to turn trustingly to the therapist, based on an isolated positive experience with the grandpa for example. This is then referred to as a mild idealizing transference. If this is not the case at all, the mistrust is sometimes so great that therapeutic relationships can very quickly be perceived as threatening and insufficient. Therapies are then terminated prematurely due to this too negative transference.

Example

A patient who had received little time and attention from her parents was often sent to her mother's parents. There she felt accepted and could literally "soak up" the warmth and understanding of the grandparents. Another patient, on the other hand, went from the frying pan into the fire: the grandparents were stricter than her own parents and demanded even more subordination and adaptation. Eventually, there was even abuse by the grandfather. ◄

3.4 Peers—The Group of Same-Aged Individuals

As we have seen, contacts usually become more diverse and complex from early childhood onwards. By the time of school enrollment at the latest, a point at which a certain cognitive and emotional maturity should be present, the social structure in which a child is integrated is already established in important basic features. Many patients report in preliminary discussions that they were already shy and sensitive people at this age, finding it difficult to establish contacts with previously unknown people. The background to such developments, which can be seen as depression already in childhood, are usually problems of the parents with their own lifestyle. Thus, fathers and mothers who are themselves preoccupied with their own emotional issues have less inner space available to respond resonantly to the emotionality and needs of their children. These children then feel emotionally abandoned and usually withdraw from disappointing and hurtful contacts.

Sometimes it is possible to compensate for these developments to some extent through warm contact with another relative such as a grandparent, resulting in less severe courses and better prognoses. The constant concern for the well-being of at least one parent is contrasted by the children's inner withdrawal in families with a lot of conflict and underlying tensions. Professionals then speak of parentification, the attempt at "parenting", caring for parents perceived as overwhelmed. This in turn overwhelms the children, so that a vicious circle can develop.

Difficulties in Gradual Detachment

The main aspect against our background of considering development in group contexts, however, is that children who are negatively (usually insecure-avoidant) attached to their parents are less able to detach from them. They are constantly connected to them with worry. The care for the parents naturally also stems from the understandable hope of eventually receiving the attention one needs. If the parents were doing well, so would one. Thus, one encounters children who have few friends at the time of school enrollment, are very anxious and only focused on the immediate family. Others, on the other hand, have already expanded their circles and have some friends, sometimes a first circle of friends, regular meetings, joint activities, either organized by the parents or in clubs. This becomes all the more significant as starting school is a psychological challenge for children: they are expected to position themselves in a larger group (class), preferably not to fall into a scapegoat role, to balance their needs and those of others, all of these complex processes in which, of course, the teachers and parents are still very often asked as moderators and decision-makers. Thus, starting school itself is an extremely differently experienced event. What for some possesses a certain anticipation and self-evidence, is for others fear-inducing and full of unknown variables. As is known from group therapy, the initial situation of a group in general, here also the entry into a new, just constituting group (the school class), is particularly tricky. Here, massive anxiety-related reactions and fears of loss, also fears of being flooded by otherwise blocked inner feelings and images can occur. When people start a psychotherapeutic group, exactly these fears experienced in childhood, such as the fear of surrender, of verbal or physical attacks, of shame and also of narcissistic damage can be reactivated and lead to intense emotional reactions at the beginning, which usually arrive devaluing and shame-triggering at the others. Here, the leader or participants with positively toned prior experience in groups are needed.

3.5 Latency Period

From a classical psychoanalytic perspective, the time between school enrollment age and the onset of puberty is referred to as the latency period. In this time, in the best case scenario, the first psychosocial conflicts for the child have been clarified and calmed to such an extent that it can focus on acquiring cultural techniques. The child has achieved a certain independence, ability to make contact and conflict capability, and has already built up a certain amount of self-esteem. The school institution uses this psychobiosocial background to stimulate cognitive abilities on the one hand, and on the other hand, many children at this age also start various sporting (e.g., soccer) or musical activities (learning instruments) in their free time. Although it was annoying for many people in retrospect, for many, practice forms a higher resilience and the foundations for later, more complex skills can be laid. If there are major emotional disputes within the family, the parents separate or a change of location becomes necessary for other reasons, some children soon show stress symptoms in the form of depressive or psychosomatic complaints. Often school performance declines, which can be understood as an indication of being internally absorbed with family problems. The group of origin is no longer the unit providing security and calm. It's good if alternatives have been built up by then, in the circle of peers, be it at school, in clubs, in leisure time. Then even stressful, intra-family experiences can sometimes be sufficiently well compensated.

Constant Formation of New Groups

After groups have become significant for the first time in preschool in daycare and kindergarten, it is the school class that gains psychological relevance as a large group with the start of school. Belonging to a class, and also to a specific school, contributes a lot to self-definition, just think of the widespread competitions between schools and individual classes. Teacher personalities are compared with each other and one is proud to have a "cool" teacher. Children have a very fine sense for the social background of their classmates. Personality traits are also quickly perceived and categorized. Instinctively, children group together with their peers and define the others as an "outgroup". The formation of subgroups, small groups, and friendships begins the moment children meet. Children with prominent features, whether in terms of clothing, appearance, behavior including behavior in class, are particularly noticed. The other children can then become role models on the one hand, and scapegoats and outsiders on the other, if several others agree in their perception. Arrangements for free time on afternoons or weekends arise from contacts during breaks or on the way to school. In physical education, the unconscious rules of group formation ensure that competition develops and the strengthening of each individual group is developed. Something like a group identity is created. While school classes are externally determined groups, students choose their friends from these groups in personal contact, so that overlapping subgroups also form. The social structure within and between the groups, but also their reflection in the individual child, gradually becomes more complex and multi-layered.

The Social Self

Looking at the events from the group perspective between the start of school and the onset of puberty, it becomes clear that beyond learning materials and performance stress, the most important thing is always happening on the side: the development of the social self. Especially in the "free" times beyond obligations through lessons and homework, children meet each other by free choice. Especially in the somewhat freer context of sports clubs, in football teams, teams and later interest-led working groups within the school, adolescents are challenged to determine, mark and enforce their social position. The prevailing customs and the choice of communication tools for the past 15 years determine the codes with which one comes into contact with each other. If someone falls too far out of the frame of these accepted social codes, it can quickly lead to the exclusion of non-conformists. The strong social pressure that children are exposed to and which they are often inclined to pass on without reflection becomes particularly visible here. The convergence to the middle, to the "that's normal", is particularly pronounced at this time. In puberty, the picture differentiates again, here "eccentrics" become more acceptable and "odd birds" can gain popularity, as opposition to parental and thus societal guidelines becomes more popular. The fact that a lot is about school grades and learning material in latency. But this is already being relativized again in its one-sidedness, shown by the fact that many children start to devote themselves to a sport or also to learning a musical instrument.

Striving for Adaptation and Differentiation

In addition to the general, the adaptation to the performance level in the class, the aim is to differentiate oneself, to discover and cultivate one's own strengths beyond the required measure. That this requires stimulation is obvious. The social background plays a major role in the selection of activities. The acquisition of these so-called cultural techniques is very important insofar as they allow one to do something for one's self-confidence, to find a vent for self-expression, also in the emotional area and last but not least: to find a group identity and to experience it. The perceived belonging and the knowledge about the importance that one has for the football or hockey team, for the orchestra, promote the awareness of one's own role in the social environment and also the relativity of one's own position. There are always others there who also attract attention. One is challenged to process and express emotions such as envy, ambition, jealousy, pride, and disappointment appropriately. In this respect, the social relationships built up in this way always also act as a corrective against narcissistic tendencies. This development points to a paradox: one does not take oneself so seriously because one is part of a larger whole. Nevertheless, one's own importance arises from the specific function for a larger group. Examples such as the sports team can show well how social groups, here based on a rule-guided sport, come together and give the individual support and security. This shows the interweaving of the levels of individuals and groups, as described by Dalal (1998).

Reflection of Personal Abilities and Characteristics

The experience that one's own abilities and skills, whether they are intellectual, physical, or musical in nature, can be expressed and that they find recognition and resonance, is fundamental for the development of a healthy self-esteem. The relationship with parents alone would be overwhelmed by this. The social environment gains more weight, can do significantly more than the nuclear family alone. This also applies to the situation of children who grow up with a single or divorced parent, sometimes in blended families. The larger group of an extended family is only maintained in rarer cases and even less often is lived together. Especially in rural areas, however, family cohesion is still stronger than in large cities. What will keep us busy again and again is that our identity is shaped by many overlapping group affiliations. These are also constantly changing. This can also lead to internal conflicts when the groups themselves define themselves more by demarcation. Contrary values in the different groups can then trigger internal dynamics. So it can happen that one has to justify oneself if one practices martial arts on the one hand, but learns to play the harp on the other. Environmental activism might not go down too well in an environment that is used to making expensive trips. Here, people of all ages are constantly faced with the question of what is more important to them personally. Not all group affiliations are always compatible with this.

3.6 Destructiveness in the Family

When there are strong burdens on the children in the family due to alcoholism and mental health problems, the circle of friends becomes increasingly important for some. The search for an "alternative family" leads, for example, to children trying to extend the time they spend in their friends' families: they stay for dinner, they go on vacation with the other family. The worse the situation in the family of origin, the less parents react to these signs from the children. Often they are also unfortunately not able to change their behavior. Children with alcoholic parents find their "chosen family" outside and can sometimes develop astonishing resilience.

Example

A patient recounted how important it had been for her to often be taken along on vacation by her best friend's family. Here she experienced relatedness, common (family) rituals, and a resilient, conflict-capable togetherness. This also helped her to better endure it at home: She was always driven by the hope of having it better or doing better one day. Thus, the other family, which nevertheless also made her envious, ensured that she developed resources to move forward in her life and to be a better mother to her daughter. Nevertheless, she still struggled with the feeling of being short-changed even in adulthood. ◄

References

Bärfuss, L (2022) Vaters Kiste. Eine Geschichte über das Erben. Rowohlt, Hamburg
Bode, S (2004) Die vergessene Generation. Klett-Cotta, Stuttgart

Dalal, F (1998) Taking the group seriously. Jessica Kingsley Publishers, London
Geyer, M (2023) Die Gruppe als normative Instanz im Wandel der Zeiten. Gruppenpsychother. Gruppendynamik 59: 1, 2–16
Grieser, J (2015) Triangulierung. Psychosozial-Verlag, Gießen
Grossmann, K E, Grossmann, K (2015) Bindung und menschliche Entwicklung. Klett-Cotta, Stuttgart
Hillman, J (2002) Charakter und Bestimmung. Goldmann, München
Kalsched, D (1996) The Inner World of Trauma. Routledge, London
Lorenz, H (2021) Die Akte Verschickungskinder. Beltz, Weinheim
Lorenz, H (2003) Kriegskinder. List, Berlin
Mitscherlich, A, Mitscherlich-Nielsen, M (1985) Die Unfähigkeit zu trauern. Fischer, Frankfurt/M
Neumann, E (1993) Tiefenpsychologie und neue Ethik. Fischer, Frankfurt/M
Nitsun, M (2014) The Anti-Group. Routledge, London
Roehler, O (2020) Der Mangel. Ullstein, Berlin
Röhl, A (2022) Das Elend der Verschickungskinder. Psychosozial-Verlag, Gießen
Sloterdijk, P (1998) Sphären: Blasen. Suhrkamp, Frankfurt/M
Wilke, G (2017) Ordnung und Chaos in Gruppen. LIT, Münster
Winnicott, D W (1960) The theory of the parent-infant relationship. International Journal of Psychoanalysis, 41: 585–595
Winnicott, D W (1974) Ichverzerrung in Form des wahren und des falschen Selbst. In: Reifungsprozesse und fördernde Umwelt. S. Fischer, Frankfurt/M, 182–199

4 Youth

Abstract

We examine the profound conflicts that can resurface during adolescence. Even during this time, when the adult personality begins to develop, when deep upheavals occur and previously held certainties about life are tested in disconcerting ways, it is always also about connecting to groups. The peer group as a "second family" can help cushion the gradual separation from the parental home and family of origin. Some seem torn between the desires for the continuation of being cared for as a child and the desire for breakout and conquering the world. Some can only endure this by occasionally escaping into dream worlds and numbing themselves.

Physical and psychological changes

The most important characteristic of adolescence is the profound psychological changes brought about by the physical and emotional maturation process of puberty. Nothing is as challenging, confusing, and exciting in a positive sense for adolescents themselves, but also for their parents, as the transformation that turns children into adults. This process varies for each individual. There is a considerable range of variation in both the speed and the breadth and depth of the effects. Often it is difficult to say where the boundary lies between still difficult but manageable crisis manifestations and a manifest psychological abnormality. In any case, this phase of life leaves no one cold and usually all those involved are glad when it is over.

The most striking feature of this developmental phase is the sexual maturation caused by hormonal changes and the emerging interest in sexuality. This is a not to be underestimated adjustment that poses new challenges for adolescents. In addition to the maturation of the body, which can cause various dissatisfactions, the interest is largely focused on the question of how to make contact with the desired

V. Münch, *Group Experience as a Resource*,
https://doi.org/10.1007/978-3-662-70864-4_4

sex without the risk of embarrassment or rejection becoming too strong. A major role is played by whether adolescents at this time are integrated into a stable, functioning network of friends and acquaintances. And whether they were able to build a resilient self-esteem in their childhood. The new desires and frustrations can thus be better absorbed than is the case when children at the end of the latency period have already spent a lot of time alone or in front of some screen.

Early partner relationships as an attempt at detachment
The psychological structures built up to this point, in which both learned skills and abilities as well as emotional maturity and bonding experiences are reflected, are crucial for the way the coming years will be experienced. Especially lonely children at the beginning of puberty run the risk of "disappearing" very early into pair relationships and sexuality, seeking their unfulfilled longings for acceptance and relief in these. But in doing so, they once again lose their group-relatedness and the chance to ally themselves with the group of peers in order to have a kind of secondary family experience. Couples are viewed suspiciously by groups, as the energy emanating from couples, especially from newly in love ones (according to the motto "we two against the rest of the world"), seems to no longer need the group as a protective and connecting place with the world of many. So a mutual aversion quickly arises, on the one hand of the group towards the "dallying two", on the other hand the couple may quickly be content with themselves. Ultimately, this process of course represents a regression at its core, which would be temporarily unproblematic, but in the long term rejects the invitation to triangulation at a new level contained therein.

Bion's basic assumption groups
Bion (1991) attributed a comparatively mature coping mode to the so-called pair formation group in his concept of basic assumption groups. He associated this defense mode against regressive fears with the oedipal fantasy about the group leader couple. These assumptions are of course also applicable to any other group, such as the often unstructured and loose groups of adolescents (called "cliques" by boomers). Also two group participants who join together in these groups, from the moment they behave as a couple or otherwise mark this, have a different position in the group. The group will tend to be skeptical, as the two "defectors" from this point on are no longer dependent on the group to the same extent and may not behave loyally towards it alone. Therefore, when a pair formation occurs, there is usually a noticeable emotional withdrawal of the other group participants.

It is the privilege of youth to enter into and dissolve many possible connections during this time in a playful way and without severe humiliation or loss experiences. But if the object experiences in the previous course of life have not gone too well, there is a greatly increased risk of renewed disappointment. Therefore, the first lasting relationships are also of interest. In my anamneses, I always ask in detail about how the first intimate relationship went and how it ended. If bad separations have happened here and severe injuries have occurred, it may be that the current problems of adult patients still have something to do with these unprocessed situations. The first great love is an important relationship in the life of every human being. And of course it refers to early childhood, when other first great loves like the mother or father played a bigger role. A rule of thumb says that the problems that were left in childhood and were not processed become a topic again about 10 years later: in the relationships of adolescents to their partners and also still to their parents.

Couples and Groups
However, couples also need groups to remain stable in the long term. Contacts with people outside of a dyad are essential to establish a balance. No person can satisfy another in everything. There are always conflicts and inadequacies that are easier to discuss with a friend. And all problems are rarely discussable with the *one* partner. But if there is the unspoken claim that this should be the case—an idealization of the couple relationship, which is not so rare in our culture (cf. Illouz 2016)—then couples put themselves under unnecessary stress and overburden the relationship. The distance that is otherwise established by the "external contacts" of the dyad may then only be achieved again through a factual separation. The longing *for* and the simultaneous fear *of* the merging of two people has led to the realization that life as a couple is made too difficult. There are indeed many patients, many also with an oedipal conflict situation, often children of divorce, who preserve an idealized image of the mostly opposite-sex parent and project it onto their partners. If it turns out that the partner cannot meet these demands, it becomes difficult. Sometimes this leads to a seemingly endless series of attempts to enter into a successful partnership. In the libretto of the opera "La Boheme", Marcello says to the idealizing Rodolfo about his love for Musetta in the sense: "I don't take love so seriously, then it can succeed better." Whoever does not demand everything from another can be less disappointed. Whoever has too high ideal notions of *the* one, all-fulfilling love, can fail more easily.

Example

A 35-year-old patient reported frequently changing relationships with women, he always ended up with women who struggled with life management. He quickly got involved, including sexually, and then often felt emotionally overwhelmed. This led him taking many steps too quickly. Once they moved in together after 3 months, and after another 3 months the love ended and they cleared out the apartment. The high emotional and also financial and organizational price that the patient was willing to pay for his attempt to enter into a secure relationship for him is the problem: Behind this is his lack of ability to care for himself, which also showed in a too low tolerance for tension and the lack of ability to critically review his own emotional situation. This always led to the same situation and the same outcome. The high importance that the patient also gave to sexuality within the relationship caused the other aspects to lose focus and also led him to come together with partners who also suffered from an attachment disorder, which they tried to solve sexually. ◄

One aspect in difficult partner relationships, as they can manifest for the first time more clearly in puberty, are the insufficiently resolved problematic attachment patterns in relation to mother or father. Men bound to their mother in this way tend to take great care of their partners' problems, and this constellation also exists the other way around. The pattern of childlike emotional deprivation, which can be found in almost all patient stories, has led to parentification: As a child, and even more so later in their partnerships, they try to help their parents and then their partners out of their perceived misery, usually disregarding their own needs and desires. These are put aside and a considerable potential for neediness and resentment accumulates, which usually remains very unconscious. The unconscious, underlying tension then leads to frequent arguments and disputes in new relationships.

4.1 Regression in the Group

Teenagers have always been enthusiastic about music and the ability to experience it live and in large groups. Just last summer, several younger participants of my group therapies were at festivals. They reported trance-like states that the constant sound and drug use had on them. To relax from relaxing, these large events had "chill-rooms" where you could regulate yourself down by lying on sofas with quieter music from headphones. The other group participants and I, of course also had critical comments at hand, but at this point I wanted to leave and acknowledge the desire for certain, culturally accepted forms of regression. If we are honest, then most people have sought out such retreats and gained experiences in their youth. Over the years, the frequency and intensity of music- and drug-induced or -accompanied excesses of this kind decrease, group experiences of this kind such as large events are less frequently visited. Why is that? Two alternative, perhaps complementary, explanatory approaches:

Music Consumption as Resource Activation

On the one hand, adolescence represents an unprecedented time of internal changes and challenges, leading to considerable uncertainty. To cope with this, those affected must constantly reassure themselves, essentially taking an emotional break to gradually get used to the exposure of adulthood. Regressive, nurturing illusions are reactivated, reminding of effortless phases of development and potentially conveying confidence and self-assurance. In line with a quasi-automated resource orientation, memories that can evoke positive feelings are recalled. The de-individualizing property of large groups under the influence of a central force (music, ideology, body self-experience) temporarily relieves the individual from the tensions and conflicts of the individual life situation. In more mature years, this relief option shifts towards other modes. These include developments towards addiction-like escape attempts (smoking, drinking, work addiction, pornography addiction, etc.) or more constructive coping modes such as activities in sports, art, music, or meditation. The great longing for security in youth due to uncertainty is partially answered in adulthood: either one feels comfortable in contact with their family, or one has otherwise settled in their life. The longing for transient regression finds a more diverse and subtle expression.

Benign Regression in Later Life

The other idea regarding why mass events like festivals are generally not attended as numerously by older people would be a decreasing ability for imagination, regression, physical-emotional exceptional states. With increasing age, the defense against emotional distress becomes increasingly routine and is also reflected in the basic physical tension. The former openness fades, one becomes slower, more cumbersome, less permeable. To cope with everyday life, this is partly a necessity and a welcome structuring. In Analytical Psychology, this would be referred to as a hypertrophy of the ego. Building a life, pursuing professional and private goals requires a price. However, to allow the regression outlined above, a greater openness towards oneself is needed. But this has become more dangerous over the years, as most people's defense has learned to successfully ward off intrusions from this area to be safe from surprises in everyday life. Only towards midlife (cf. Münch 2016) such shocks become more frequent again, when the price of repressing regressive impulses has become too high. Then often psychosomatic and depressive symptom formations show. Also in psychotherapies, it is precisely about this: that a greater openness towards unconscious life is achieved and repressed emotions, dreams, and areas of experience become more conscious again. What midlife and the then visible limits of conscious goal setting remind us of is that structure and success are always only one side of the coin. The other side is the price that repression and avoidance can have. Most treatments are about accepting the unavailable, about being able to let go, about humility, about a physical "softening", about being able to allow feelings like fear, shame, guilt, worry, pain, and grief again. Put differently, it is about the acceptance of perceived weaknesses leading to real authenticity, to inner strength. Individuation, the development towards what I experience as authentic and belonging to me, is a process that is partly directed against societal currents, against others. At the same time, we always draw from the fund of the surrounding culture in the process of this self-realization. Absolute autonomy and distinguishability is an illusion, there are always intersections of our personality with that of others. And here we see that we are already back in the midst of group experiences.

Example

Patients who could only follow their own paths to a small extent in their youth, who were too much at the mercy of the projections of their caregivers, often show very little reference to what we as therapists understand as the "true self" in the sense of Winnicott. This usually reflects an early experience with the first caregiver. Time and again, patients who have remained very dependent overall in middle age tell me that they still call their "mom" every day. For some, she lives in the same house, so they cross paths every day. It turned out that any demarcation or criticism was frowned upon, the mom was the best friend, after all, she had already adopted the hobbies and interests of usually the daughter during puberty. The patients then reported joint concert visits and trips. It would not have been my job to interpret all this, had there not often been massive psychosomatic complaints, divorces, workplace problems (due to lack of demarcation!). ◄

4.2 The Second Family

If one fails to establish a "second family" in the form of a peer group, where the values that were previously considered significant and unquestionable can be viewed more distantly, then someone remains bound to their early objects. At this developmental threshold, significant humiliations often occur, driving individuals back to parental figures for comfort. The initially strange behavior of many joint activities with parents often arises from the need not to be able to break into the world of objects outside the protective family. This leads to a neurotic compromise: the conquest of something new in the outside world, but in the company of the parental figure. This process cannot naturally lead to detachment. The dynamic background is usually that the ego of the patients is not securely bound and inevitable frustrations in the course of the sometimes unimaginable separation or moving out of home cannot be processed constructively. The move back in with the parents (usually only to the preferred parent) indicates that there are still great desires and longings for care and security, without whose fulfillment no detachment seems possible. I think of a patient who had gone through and suffered this back and forth of moving out and moving back in many times.

Repeated Triangulation Steps

Let's take a step back. Since the phase of early puberty is primarily about another triangulation, it is significant whether similar processes have already taken place in a favorable, development-promoting sense in early childhood or whether development is arrested because this was not the case. Often the dynamics repeat themselves on a new level and with an even greater amplitude. If the ability to triangulate is overwhelmed, for example due to a divorce of the parents, a problematic development can also result. The affected individuals are not capable of further psychological maturation. Children of single parents can get into the conflict that they cannot leave the single parent alone on the one hand, but would like to pursue their own interests increasingly on the other hand. This often leads to panic disorders and identity crises, especially in sons of rather depressive mothers. One patient was suddenly dropped by her clique for a minor thing in her youth. This triggered a retreat to her parents' house and practically erased the previously achieved steps of individuation. Only in the school area did the patient still "function". Internally, however, she had given up all hope of a truly independent life.

Every clique of adolescent friends has its own rules and codes. It is very important for adolescents whether they find contact with such a group, otherwise they lack an important element for their further internal development. Before entering adulthood, there are several developmentally relevant, but also simultaneously vulnerable phases, in which making contact with non-family others is easier for many than in other life phases. This concerns early childhood around the 4th year of life, 10 years later early puberty and, in my opinion, also for some shortly after studies and training, about 24. Important internal structures are formed on the basis of the contacts and bonds experienced then. If there are already early developmental arrests, it is also more likely that the corresponding puberty time will also be problematic. The group of peers, whether loosely composed or consisting of classmates or training or study colleagues, can help initiate the internal and later also the external farewell to the parents' house.

Example

A 30-year-old patient had lived with his mother until recently. He was an only child and his mother had separated from his father early on. In his own apartment, he soon had panic attacks and then sought therapeutic help. It turned out that he had no image of himself as a man and his self-assertion and aggression were very inhibited. During the course of treatment, he also visited a men's group, which provided him with important suggestions. Gradually, his handling of his feelings, his coping with reality, and his symptoms improved. Eventually, he found a girlfriend. ◄

The highly stimulated fantasy life in puberty, the significance that sexuality gains for mental life,—all this leads in the case of fewer concrete experiences in and with groups of peers or slightly older people to an increasing "escape from reality". Currently, this dynamic is usually reflected in the fact that teenagers are engaged in (online) computer games for hours and days on end. In the virtual worlds, they find the heroes and adventures that real life does not offer. Here, something is often playfully played out that can be understood as an attempt at initiation, something that is seen in society as having little significance. An internal too strong "escape from reality" often remains unnoticed at first, either because it is assumed that the teenagers will give up their withdrawn behavior after a corresponding "phase"; or because the hidden construction of grandiose fantasies is seen as a sign of the ongoing internal emancipation of the teenager. Mind you: it is about the interpretation of the behavior of teenagers by their reference persons. In many treatments with patients who have grown older in this way, it only comes to light late how they had equipped their internal self-esteem with unconscious grandiose ideas, as they largely lacked real reinforcing experiences.

Example

A patient came into inpatient treatment after his high school graduation, having already reacted for months with severe social withdrawal, tension, sleep disorders, and panic attacks with agoraphobia (fear of open spaces). He had little connection to his self and showed great confusion and overwhelm in the face of normal social situations, especially in groups. After his hospital stay, he began attending an outpatient analytical group on advice, which he visited for several years. Here, for the first time, he was able to build communication and attachment to others in a protected setting and in a reflective manner mirrored by others. It turned out that it was completely unfamiliar to him that other people mirrored his behavior. Neither parents nor peers had seriously undertaken this. ◄

Of course, there are also group members in group psychotherapies who have managed to make positive and emancipatory experiences after perhaps more difficult early childhood socialization experiences in their youth. Thus, they can help others in a group regain their hope. Each participant in each group is at a different inner place at a given time, holds a different psychological position. This affects the others in such a way that identifications can form, that structural gaps can be closed through interactions, in short, that more trusting human bonds can be built. The diversity of people is helpful because they can help each other at different points, because they each have something "ahead" of the others.

Example

A patient who had experienced multiple sexual assaults in her late adolescence struggled in her relationship and at work with articulating her own desires and positions. Even in front of the group she later joined, she hid these experiences for a long time. But in doing so, she repeated her silent and passive behavior towards the group. In her unconscious staging, the group became the insensitive, potentially rejecting counterpart. Only gradually was she able to give up this resistance and stand up for herself more by first talking about it in the parallel individual sessions. ◄

Groups of Like-minded People

I would like to call those virtual groups "groups in spirit" that children already join to exchange ideas, play together, chat, communicate. We all saw in April 2023 what can happen when young adults stand out in a chat group and want to show off. Here it was a 21-year-old military member who posted secrets of the US government about the background of the Ukraine war in a forum. Another phenomenon, especially important in adolescence, is the widespread distribution of pornography. Similar to dealing with other internet content, it is crucial what personal stability and bonding experience the individuals have. Especially teenagers without satisfying and close (friendship) relationships, but also those with a conflict-ridden parent relationship, are more at risk of consuming pornographic content in an addictive manner to stabilize their inner balance and self-esteem. Non-sexual needs are then tried to be compensated through the sexualized fantasy life. The problem is again the virtuality of the experience: essentially beautiful experiences are only made in the fantasy and with one's own body, cannot be understood and integrated with real people and within a relationship. Thus, they lead a split existence in soul's life, are also harder to influence. But it should be like that: Wilhelm (2023) writes that "the group … becomes more important than the I, … when individuals define their self-concept through the group and identify with it" (p. 35). That individual needs and identity features can recede behind group identification is not only a characteristic of group phenomena in adolescence.

4.3 Once again: School, Leisure and Interests

Puberty as the time of reaching sexual maturity and adolescence as the time of internal mental maturation to adulthood go hand in hand. Similarly, the often rather exclusive contrast between leisure interests and career aspirations is also the case. The still playful and experimental approach to one's own talents, abilities and curiosity is of great importance. Those who feel compelled to commit themselves too early to a profession or training, measured against their own willingness to do so, are likely to feel the need to reconsider this decision later on. Again and again, I have encountered patients who, having grown up in a rather educationally distant, action-oriented milieu, initially learned a vocational profession (such as carpenter, hairdresser, educator). A decade later or often in midlife around forty, first doubts or health problems arose and some began retraining, applying for other jobs. Normally, during my childhood and adolescence, I notice what interests I have, what excites and attracts me. Here, the reflection by parents or teachers plays a major role. Some of this turns out to be unattainable for me, either because abilities are lacking or because the motivation to perform, the ambition is lacking. Many of these initially childish wishes are later modified or abandoned. Those who experience being entrusted with responsibility in certain areas of life (such as in sports or youth groups), those who experience that their mentor or teacher support and believe in them, in them the conviction solidifies that they can believe in themselves. As well, a musical performance also takes place in a class and in front of a group of interested people, including hopefully the own parents. Always a child learns implicitly that it is part of a group, a larger unit of people. Over time, this determines more precisely where one's own place in society is, where one wishes to be and what will probably never be possible.

The Downsides of Homeschooling and Home Office

Schoolchildren got an unpleasant taste of the world of home office in the post-Covid-19 world during the so-called homeschooling in the years of the coronavirus pandemic. Also, the compulsion for parents to have to do their work from home on the computer and no longer be able to experience interruptions through personal encounters in the hallway, in the break room, when getting coffee, etc., led to an increase in their complaints in many of my depressive patients! Especially socially relatively isolated people experienced it as extremely restrictive and frustrating to be deprived of this opportunity for physical encounter. The lack of eye contact, the limited frequency of the voice, the "intangibility" of the other hurts many. In this respect, it is also about the enrichment and the developmental promoting function of groups: school classes, circles of friends and work colleagues are, even if they can sometimes be annoying, essential for the personality development of people. This works primarily live, in presence, as it also requires lively visual, auditory, haptic and olfactory exchange. In this respect, personal contact in its diversity is the most important criterion for healthy mental development in adolescence. During the pandemic, the worlds of children, adolescents and adults met unintentionally: everyone had to work from home. Some in homeschooling and others in the home office. The development of inner spaces was also hindered by the closure of outer spaces, an unusually large number of adolescents had to undergo psychiatric and psychotherapeutic treatment.

Especially the stress that entered many families, especially underprivileged ones, shows how important it is to be able to retreat into one's school or professional groups. The developmentally necessary retreat of adolescents was in danger. This also leads to the insight that school and training is only partly about the transmission of knowledge, work is only partly about productivity and performance. It is always also about the socially important interweaving of individuals into groups and the exchange between them. Without this experience, we would not be able to live. This is increasingly being neglected in our strongly individualistic worldview. Especially the hype about the possibilities of digital tools makes these arguments less and less valid. I repeat myself: It is crucial whether a teenager has internalized positive social experiences as a child. Then he can unscathed experience a phase of "diving", for example into PC games or other virtual escapades. Also as long as there are currently enough real relationships, real experiences, either in internalized form, which means mental structure, or in perhaps few, but sustainable personal contacts in the real world outside the digital bubble, there is usually no great cause for concern. However, parents should accompany the development of their children as best they can and confront them if necessary, if parental rules are no longer being followed at all.

Example

A young man, who had been supported by his parents in his musical interests all his life and had become very successful with it, questioned his own development. He thought that he would probably have taken a completely different path if he had not also been pushed again and again. Internally, he was strongly bound to his mother through his history, and he had very ambivalent feelings towards his father. After a longer therapy, he met a woman with whom he could find a new togetherness, after he had often fought in vain for the affection of women before. He was able to let go of the desire to be understood by his mother and thus opened up new possibilities for himself. ◄

4.4 Bad Company

With the choice of friends and peers, adolescents show what and who is really important to them. Their inner world is reflected in their surroundings. This may frighten parents, but it deserves attention. If we assume that not only the choice of partner, but also the selection of friends is not only driven by the compulsion to repeat, i.e., the selection oriented towards the parents' model, but also brings to light hitherto dormant aspects of the personalities of the people concerned, then the question of which group someone forms around themselves in their youth (not only which other groups he or she joins) takes on a new meaning. The inner groupality (Kaes) or the dissociability of the psyche (Jung) finds its correspondence in the sometimes inhomogeneous, sometimes alienating circles of friends. Who am I and if so, how many, is a question particularly often asked by young people, who hopefully have the opportunity to discover and develop as many and perhaps sometimes contradictory parts of themselves in others (cf. Precht, 2011).

Innate Talents and Tendencies
Hillman (2002) emphasizes that a child's talents need not be learned or biographically anchored. Discovering and respecting them, thinking of child development not as ideal-typical and schematic and also malleable, questions many notions of education and pedagogy. If one takes seriously what the author elaborates, then new ideas and creativity can only emerge when there is the freedom to behave inappropriately and act against the expectations of the environment. This points to originality and authenticity. Children usually choose the groups that suit them. The identification sought there can have something strengthening and inspiring.

However, this can also lead to problematic developments if a too sharp demarcation is sought, if much suppressed aggression against subjectively perceived, years-long suppression of one's own needs is expressed in it. This can then manifest itself as delinquency or drug abuse. However, most adolescents manage to rein in and get a grip on behavioral problems after their youth. Normally, the family of origin gradually lets go of the adolescents during this time and thus hands over more self-responsibility to them. However, it seems essential that the self-parts that came to life as a child must be saved over the time of youth. The connection between the vital self-expressions of the child, his dreams and the joy of self-discoveries is ideally transferred to the activities of youth and then later transformed into the choice of a profession.

4.5 Training and Student Groups

4.5.1 Education

Adolescents who start an apprenticeship after their secondary school graduation usually still live at their parents' home. For cost reasons and because they are rarely of age yet. With the training, they come into an environment that demands a profound restructuring of their daily routine and their living environment. On the other hand, they get the chance to develop their abilities and talents and to experience that self-discipline and diligence pay off for them. Depending on how far the other social development has already progressed, the known problems occur. If heartache and romantic exuberance rule, the training or further school education can also be affected. Especially the tension between what is already demanded in terms of self-discipline, what unresolved conflicts arise from tensions with parents, which good or disappointing experiences are made in connection with first love, can result in a melange of strongly contradictory feelings and an incoherent self-image, which sometimes manifests itself in displacement actions. Then there is excessive substance abuse, mental difficulties or strong self-doubts and disorientation. Conflicts with authority figures such as teachers or superiors often repeat or double if the conflicts with the parents are not resolved. It would then be helpful to be integrated into a third group such as a club (e.g., sports) or a community (e.g., parish), where third parties can have a mediating or calming effect.

Example

A now over 40-year-old patient had already had major conflicts in his parents' home as a teenager and young adult. The resulting regular cannabis use lasted for many years. To this day, the patient cannot restore contact with his parents except for brief moments, as he feels unrecognized by them and this would seem like self-betrayal to him. Out of defensive reasons, he has put himself into a kind of timeless state that allows few changes and little development. To stand against the parents means for him to exclude the real parents from his life. This indicates that the inner parental images still oppress him too much and are too close to him. It is to be assumed that a separation could not be adequately carried out for him at different levels and at different times of life as a child, teenager and adult, as too little self-esteem has arisen due to the parents described as intrusive. Paradoxically, separation can only be experienced through the feeling of being "against" the parents. But with this, he remains strongly connected to them internally. ◄

4.5.2 Studies

Even young adults who start studying after graduating from high school often live with their parents more frequently than before. On the other hand, they often form new groups with acquaintances, friends, and fellow students and establish a shared living community. This also reflects the tendency towards group formation. In these shared living communities, mutual stimulation, community, and sometimes even the exploration of new life models are sought. Unconsciously, for some, the dynamics of childhood can repeat themselves in these communities. Especially those who hope for harmonious coexistence inmany communal activities can be disappointed when the roommates pursue their own goals. Interesting in the group context is also the more frequent observation that those who imagine a “counter-model” to the model experienced in childhood identify with very similar authoritarian structures as those they reject. The identification with the aggressor, i.e., the perpetrator introject, obscures the view, regardless of whether the ideological and social goals and ideals of the persons concerned can now be completely different. The form seems to dominate the content here.

Steinmayr (2023) describes the changed perception of teaching. Today, the university is largely seen as a service company that owes something to its students. The author is concerned that the idea of science is less conveyed than its contents. He interprets universities primarily “as a place where the dialogue of generations takes place”, it is about a “mutual listening to each other and learning from each other” (p. 15). The development he observed also suggests that the potential and resources of groups are used less today than in the past. This also closes the circle to criticism of virtual forums, which are mainly perceived when they provide a platform for a “shitstorm”. The term “milieu”, to which Steinmayr also refers, seems to have completely gone out of fashion: a student milieu, hardly anyone talks about it today. Studying as a phase of life in which one can try out different models of life and weigh up views on life against each other—all this has increasingly receded into the background in the face of Bologna reforms, performance pressure, and high financial pressure.

Trying out new forms of life

The experimentation with new forms of life in student circles, including the so-called “free love”, now referred to as “polyamory”, as it was already tried out in “communes” 60 years ago and led to injuries and frustrations, also involves the revival of apparently unresolved ambivalences of fathers, mothers, and grandparents. The movement seems to oscillate between a search and curiosity movement on the one hand and a disappointed retreat from too high ideals on the other. This affects both the forms of cohabitation and the variations of what we call love. Erotic freedom is once again assigned a higher value. This can be understood as hedonism or as an attempt to liberate oneself from norms, but in any case as an effort to differentiate oneself. Many people want to try something out to see what it does to them. They are less concerned with an apodictic ideology than with the search for what is consistent and suitable for them in relationship matters, but above all what is livable. Not a few ultimately fail due to their persistent feelings of jealousy or fear of abandonment, they then slowly approach the long-avoided or conflict-ridden parental forms of life. Others seem unable to do this and continue to search for the right form of life for them. Each generation must find its own truth and balance and be allowed to put old certainties and traditional forms of life to the test. It is always about trying out where one stands, where one belongs, with which others one can relate in agreement. Where is an exchange? Where is the group to which I mean something and which gives me support? Are there others who feel the same way as I do? Am I also allowed to break away from the group? And am I still a part of it then? These are some of the significant questions at this stage of life.

References

Bion, W R (1991) Erfahrungen in Gruppen. Fischer, Frankfurt/M

Hillman, J (2002) Charakter und Bestimmung. Goldmann, München

Illouz, E (2016) Warum Liebe weh tut. Suhrkamp, Berlin

Münch, V (2016) Krise in der Lebensmitte. Springer, Heidelberg

Precht, R D (2011) Who Am I And If So, How Many? Constable, London

Steinmayr, M (2023) Zwischen Dienstleistungsdenken und Aktivismus: Universitäten in der Krise. Der Freitag 14, p. 15

Wilhelm, K (2023) Sehnsucht nach Zusammenhalt. Psychologie Heute 03/2023, 32–36. Beltz, Weinheim

5 Young Adulthood

Abstract

As young people mature into personalities, it becomes increasingly tense. Old conflicts between parents and children resurface, should they not already be resolved. New topics are added, such as the choice of partner and career. The desires to connect with groups are accompanied by the desires for a first longer intimate relationship, and it can become difficult to reconcile both. In addition, there is the still unfinished education, especially among students, and the ongoing curiosity for new experiences, which seem to contradict settling down or becoming sedentary. Many are concerned with the question of the right time for marriage, pregnancy, and starting a family. These topics are emotionally charged, especially in the case of conflict-ridden parent relationships, and sometimes hinder further development. What helpful or inhibiting influence do group dynamics have in this phase of life?

Early adulthood, which replaces adolescence for developmental psychologists (see Erikson 1973), roughly the time between the ages of 20 and 30, brings with it characteristic challenges. It is the time when the professional situation solidifies and stabilizes for some, while for others it is still a time of learning and studying. For a while, the term moratorium, a kind of grace period, was common for this. For students, despite increased performance demands and school-like curricula, it is a time of experimentation. Semesters abroad and parallel jobs as working students are common. After the biological and physical changes of puberty and the efforts of adolescence have been overcome, early adulthood cannot be completely separated from these preceding life stages. Although it is about a certain consolidation in terms of education and career as well as in private life, unresolved, unprocessed conflicts from earlier life stages can still be effective.

V. Münch, *Group Experience as a Resource*,
https://doi.org/10.1007/978-3-662-70864-4_5

The integration of even contradictory desires and emotions is already better achieved at this age than in the often turbulent youth. Depending on the predisposition, simpler or more complex processing and defense processes can help. Among these, the mechanisms of splitting off emotions or projection are certainly the least beneficial and healthy. Even young adults are still maturing in personality, which continues throughout life (see Erikson 1973). In this respect, the mentioned defense formations differ once due to the familial and other previous experiences, but also independently of this in the course of life. The ability to handle ambivalence and the integration of the emotional world and other personality parts is a lifelong process. The assumption of more extreme positions, also the feeling of clear and strong and seemingly unambiguous emotions, is rather the privilege of youth. A more differentiated view of emotions, worldviews, and opinions is only possible in the course of life through a variety of experiences and corrections in contacts.

The Shades of Gray in Life

This has also been extensively studied by the philosopher Sloterdijk (2022). He refers to the value of this increasing differentiation and distinction ability and speaks of the shades of gray in life, which initially appear colorless and not very passionate, but on closer inspection can represent a considerable variety of experiences. Without these shadow aspects, another description suggests, the bright side of life can only be appreciated a little, a situation that is rather annoying for still young contemporaries, as it has not yet occurred.

For young adults, there are some challenges at their age that are associated with the necessary establishment of an independent life. The motivation for this is generally not as great later in life. Therefore, ambitious goals are sometimes pursued, and there is considerable competition. This is mitigated by the shifting values of today's millennials. They pay more attention to a balance between work and leisure, distinguishing between the demands society places on them and the private longings and desires they have for themselves. Boomers, those over 50 today, often struggle with this changed mentality because it is so different from what they are familiar with. This can also lead to conflicts more quickly, for example, over issues of so-called work-life balance, as soon as the generations have to work together. Ultimately, this intergenerational shift in life planning priorities is something to be expected, albeit with ever new topics and favorites.

What Kind of Bonding Experience do I have?

A characteristic of early adulthood is the identity that is still fluid, but at the same time solidifying. This is not only dependent on the experiences of the family of origin, but also on later, other group experiences. We find that young adults in this age group form bonds more and more frequently. Why is this, what psychological prerequisites are at play? Those who, due to their sufficiently positive bonding experiences in childhood and adolescence, have enough ego strength, enough identity, now dare to take the step into the intimacy of a dyadic relationship (cf. Erikson 1973). In doing so, they expose themselves to the strong feelings of infatuation, sexual passion, and the tendency to idealize, all of which can have an ego-dissolving character. As a rule, this temporary regression is enjoyed and leads to inner enrichment and growth, while it can lead to insecurity, dependence, and new fears and overburdening in people with insecure self-development. Complications and conflicts in close relationships can also quickly arise under these conditions. People in their early 20s are often still very influenced by what their parents have modeled for them and relate to it. This can mean that they consciously decide against the parental "recommendations". Love partners then act like a counter-draft to the world of the parents, which can be somewhat provocative. But the opposite can also be the case: the structures of relationships then resemble those between parents and their children. This is all the more the case, the less independent the development of the children has been so far. Thus, early marriages and pregnancies occur relatively frequently when the parents themselves had already done so.

A love relationship can be experienced like diving into a new world, like crossing a border, like sharing common, just unknown experiences. Therefore, our romantic desire in particular represents a great drive to deal with the unknown, to open up to the new, the other. In other areas as well, young adults expose themselves to the influence of various, sometimes disparate groups in order to better understand themselves in the reflection through others. In any case, it is usually about very intense emotions, which are then shared in groups like circles of friends.

Example

A young patient was active in the climate protection movement and also employed at a university. To avoid disadvantages for a planned career in the civil service, he inquired in great detail about the boundaries between behavior that is not yet criminally relevant and behavior that could be assessed as a violation of boundaries and would result in an entry in the certificate of good conduct. Here we find the attempt to pursue different objectives in parallel and to minimize the disadvantages of this constellation. ◄

Many students, so my impression, have restricted their activities in the past pandemic years. Face-to-face contacts and unpredictable encounters became less frequent, contacts and appointments were planned more consciously and purposefully and sometimes even avoided. Learning formats in particular are preferred to be quickly "completed" and the practical online format is preferred. Privately, however, people prefer to meet in person. The strong focus on online formats and the semester-long impossibility of meeting in person had profound consequences for the lifestyle of a larger number of adolescents and young adults.

Example

One of my patients completely withdrew from his studies when he thought he had missed the connection. Another learned almost exclusively, avoided festive occasions and sports events, even when this was allowed again. Yet another young man suffered greatly from the under-demand in the practical phases of his dual studies as well as from the misallocation and loneliness (home office) in his job after the bachelor's degree. A home office in young adulthood therefore appears even more dysfunctional and disease-causing than this can be in later phases of life. As a rule, more people live in a shared apartment or still with their relatives and families in their 20s and are therefore less at risk of becoming lonely. ◄

There are indeed not a few adults who manage to intensify their commitments and leisure activities that began in adolescence in young adulthood. Some take on voluntary functions and help in the social sector. Others, on the other hand, withdraw from these activities and focus on learning. At this age, it becomes more noticeable that identity and self-confidence are fed to a considerable extent from belonging to several social groups. The different selection and internal weighting of the influences of these groups then make up the individuality of the persons concerned. Decisions with greater impact are required. People who were only able to establish a few individual contacts in their youth often remain alone in early adulthood, as they have fundamental problems with establishing new contacts. However, they then lack the positive experiences of feedback and also the perception of others in groups, from which one learns something about oneself. Often the affected persons then stay with the parents for a long time or sometimes only with a single parent. Thus, one also encounters people who have had no closer contact in a sexual sense even at the age of 30 and beyond. But social naivety and anxiety is sometimes also tried to be compensated by sexual overactivity. In these cases, a narcissistic problem can be assumed.

Example

A participant of my groups came to therapy at the age of 20. He felt very incapable of being alone. He repeatedly reported, fluctuating between pride and fears, about his female "conquests" and the insecurities that came with them. He was able to stabilize himself through regular physical training. Only gradually did he prove capable of maintaining a longer relationship and learning to endure inevitable frustrations. But also his ability to set boundaries and his ability to separate himself gradually increased. Slowly he discovered his own emotional position and was also better able to stand by his aversive and aggressive feelings. This eventually led to more clarity in his relationships and subsequently to more decisiveness in professional decisions. He had learned to internalize the patient and open attitude of the group towards him into his self-relationship. His aggression, which until then he had mainly directed against himself (high ego ideal), could now find its way into his actions in a more constructive way. ◄

5.1 Young Couples

Although some couples who are together in their late 20s have found each other in their youth, partnerships in the 20s of life still change relatively frequently. Of course, there is a wide range in this regard. For all couples, however, there is the psychological task of defending the newly discovered togetherness, psychologically and symbolically almost a return to the dyadic of early childhood, against the groups in the environment and at the same time staying in contact with them. This starts with the time a couple spends together. If the balance between the needs of the two partners, but also in relation to the couple and its circles of friends, leisure groups and relatives shifts and becomes too one-sided, conflicts arise. Thus, the partner who feels confronted with exaggerated demands of the other quickly feels constricted and under pressure. Some couples open their togetherness relatively quickly again to their circles of friends and thus give themselves little time to sufficiently stabilize their connection. This can then lead to premature contact with the parents of the other, which is perceived as tense. The desire for one's own parents to give their blessing to their very own decision is understandable in itself, but also paradoxical, as it can be based on a childish motivation. One wants to be independent and adult, but please with the blessing of the parents. In other words: The influence of parents on the psychological balance in patients of this age is often still large. If the professional situation is not yet clarified and the degree has not yet been achieved, this subliminally shames the children. Parents are worried and develop feelings of guilt if the children do not develop as quickly and in the direction they have envisaged for them. Everyone finds it hard to let go. Especially hard are parents whose own wishes did not play a big role at the age their children are now and who have complied with the ideas of their own parents about their future. These parents can often develop intense envy of their children and compensatorily develop a compulsion to control ("helicopter parents").

New Experiences Can Only be Made in Relationships

At the same time, people between 20 and 30 learn that relationships need time to grow. Their romantic relationships tend to become longer and more consistent. This requires a new ability to regulate. The question arises as to how one can continue to live one's own life and pursue one's friendships and interests while remaining loyal to one's relationship. Sometimes changes of location are pending due to training reasons or because of a job offer, which put a strain on the couples. In addition, as shown before, groups and couples are natural antagonists. Bion (1991) described the formation of a couple within a group as a reaction to a strong regression. Couples must be prepared for this: that their friends, the clique wants to have a say. But in these groups, one also continues to encounter others, which can sometimes make it difficult to remain faithful.

5.2 Extended Adolescent Crises

I relatively often encounter patients, especially men, who despite their age of about mid-20s seem to be in a pronounced adolescent crisis. Frequent conflicts with parents dominate their everyday life, attempts to gain a foothold and build their own life through education, studies, profession, or partnership stagnate and fail repeatedly for similar reasons. They have been enrolled in a university for a long time, they do not graduate, dissertations are abandoned. Often there is a very conflictual relationship with the father, whose life successes are doubted, who is devalued, just as he must have devalued the patients themselves in the past. These patients (I have treated many young men in this regard) seem to linger in a kind of extended adolescence. Their life seems to stand still, learning and working are procrastinated, leading to ever new feelings of guilt, which in turn are processed depressively, leading to new withdrawal and so on. It can be a great relief when these patients learn in a group to either motivate themselves anew and accept their previously unaccepted boundaries. It happens that many of these male patients, in the absence of newer acquaintances, feel very connected to their circles of friends from their youth days. Alcohol and other drugs are consumed to some extent, little is done in the friendships. Proven rituals are constantly repeated, time seems to stand still. Remaining in this group is increasingly experienced as conflictual in the course of therapy. The old buddies start to strain, one wants to develop further, the friends do not go along, do not change their behavior. Finally, the patients quit their old circle of friends.

The Influence of the Social Environment on Identity Formation
But it is very difficult to suddenly want to detach oneself completely from such a group, sometimes from an entire sociotope. This usually scares too much. Only very gradually can new interests be built up, then new contacts that can gradually replace the old ones. Group self-experience or therapy can set new accents here by allowing many different perspectives and ideas to flow in. Other participants can tell about past or current situations that are very similar, and how they have solved them. Understanding can be expressed, but also impatience and criticism. The old group loyalties are part of the identity of young adults, the first group outside the family where they felt accepted. If this has happened mainly in the context of substance abuse and generally passive behavior, then these patients will eventually catch up with their self-deception: The others, like the parents, could not really see and accept them! They have fallen into a compulsion to repeat and have not yet been able to experience anything really new.

The Concept of Emerging Adulthood

Seiffke-Krenke (2020) has made the concept of "emerging adulthood" developed by Arnett known in Germany. It describes partly problematic, partly expected developmental steps of late adolescents. These include the characteristics of extreme self-focus, increased narcissism, extension of identity development with much exploration, instability of lifestyle, predominance of (too) many options in life planning, the feeling of being "between chairs" and also the postponement of markers of adulthood. All these peculiarities can be found especially under the conditions of extended training periods, precarious employment relationships, after lack of training, but also in materially privileged circles. A certain role is certainly also played by the fact that the behavioral and lifestyle characteristics mentioned here are traded as ideal ideas and images of ideal life in popular culture well into the 4th decade. There also seems to be a convergence of previously disparate life phases. Even older people sometimes behave very youth-typically in their preferences and lifestyles.

Example

In my impression, students in the media, gaming, and film industry have established and widespread behaviors that indicate very irregular rhythms in everyday life. The ultimate goal is imagination, spontaneity, and multitasking. This leads to confusion and exhaustion in some. It can be particularly difficult to translate the high creative performance into the found formats and forms, to take care of own projects in the long term. A high degree of independence is required here, along with a high ability to open up to one's own unconscious and perceive creative impulses. The group ability of the students is often put to the test, as there is a high mutual dependency. ◄

5.3 Committing now, Having a Child Now?

Example

A young patient began studying law after various other trainings. She had fallen into a kind of mediator role due to her parents' separation, but identified more with the dominant father. However, in one point she unconsciously showed opposition to her father: While he had made a clear decision against her mother and for his second wife when she was a child, she hesitated for a long time to enter into a serious relationship. She learned to gradually confront a new partner more openly and to stand up for her needs, and thus experienced her relationship as resilient and stable. This also helped her in her studies and in shaping relationships with girlfriends, some of whom reflected the difficult mother relationship. Eventually, she got married. ◄

The fact that many people today move to more distant cities to study implies that they also fall in love and settle down there. When children are on the way, the question of care arises. The grandparents of the offspring are far away and are not spontaneously available for babysitting and other relieving support. It helps if couples, often even before they find each other, have built a network of acquaintances and friends. Studies and training, leisure and hobbies offer plenty of opportunity to build such networks. But these need to be maintained and this is not equally easy and self-evident for everyone. I keep meeting patients who find it very difficult to build contacts. They often doubt themselves, have low self-esteem and often ponder for a long time how they can approach someone. Their strict superego constantly makes them doubt themselves, their unintegrated aggression makes life difficult for them. If the opportunity has not already passed, such an appearance is of course not particularly attractive to others. This makes the matter complicated and a vicious circle.

Youth in the Digitalized World
People, or patients, who are between 18 and 25 years old at the beginning of the 2020s, know the world of communication and information largely digitalized. For them, many things about getting to know each other, communication, and also the termination of relationships present themselves differently than for previous generations. When these younger people then come together in a group with older people, different "communication worlds" collide. If the participants are open, this can be interesting for everyone, because the exchange between older (parents) and younger (children) is not always so directly possible within families. The corrective emotional experiences that the generations can collect in this regard in groups of any kind, but in a particularly intensive way in therapeutic, analytical groups, are discussed in more detail in the Chaps. 10, 11, 12 and 13. The different life backgrounds of group participants are generally a resource for everyone in a group, as this can bring a variety of alternative perspectives into consciousness. The naive assumption of those inexperienced with groups is often exactly the opposite: they assume that those working therapeutically treat disorder-specific, similarly situated "cases" together.

Example

Severely traumatized patients, such as people who grew up as an only child with alcoholic parents, can experience an alternative model for a "family", for normal interaction with each other in a group, which helps to reduce their fears in this regard. However, the hurdle of getting involved in a group at all can initially be higher due to these fears. Understandably, there is the fear that bad experiences could be repeated and thus the traumas could be touched. Very careful motivational work by the therapeutic workers is necessary here. But also training contexts that have a familial framework can have such positive effects as a group. ◄

Many students only deal with the question of whether they want to have offspring relatively late. For non-academics, it usually happens earlier. Regardless of these sociocultural differences, starting a family psychologically poses a great challenge. It takes self-confidence and courage to create a situation that can remind one of one's own childhood in many ways. Repressed unpleasant experiences can lead to the hoped-for happiness clouding over and sometimes similar dynamics as in the parental home establishing themselves. In addition to the great happiness that children mean, they also cost a lot of strength and challenge the ability to focus on the positive aspects of living together despite many de-idealizations and frustrations. Creative solutions for emerging problems are required and those who have been given little room for the development of a resilient ego in their development are particularly quickly overwhelmed.

References

Bion, W (1991) Erfahrungen in Gruppen. Fischer, Frankfurt/M

Erikson, E (1973) Identität und Lebenszyklus. Suhrkamp, Frankfurt

Seiffge-Krenke, I (2020) Weiterbildungsgebiete und Transitionsalter: Emerging Adulthood. Vortrag bei der BPtK, 24.6.2020. https://api.bptk.de/uploads/Seiffge_Krenke_B_Pt_K_Fachgespraech_Transition_240620_8511bc4d04.pdf (Stand: 17.10.2023)

Sloterdijk, P (2022) Wer noch nie Grau gedacht hat. Suhrkamp, Berlin

Midlife and the Beginning of the Second Half of Life

6

Abstract

Around so-called midlife, which is around the age of 40, many personality traits, many partnership, family, and also friendship relationships have stabilized. Naturally, this is also related to the external living conditions. Midlife is often a time for crisis-ridden developments, because stagnation threatens here and the transience of life becomes more consciously perceived. This causes fear and often motivates changes. There are developments in both directions: If one has thought too much about one's own advancement and is too little embedded in supportive groups, a more collective and connected way of life is often sought. On the other hand, if one has long hidden in "one's" groups, that is, feared one's own path of individual life design, then the psyche usually also demands to reduce this one-sidedness in favor of a more delineated and self-consistent way of life. We look at how differently singles and couples can experience this.

6.1 Midlife as a Turning Point

In Analytical Psychology, a crisis in midlife represents a significant turning point in personal, psychological development. Regardless of whether there is actually an intensification of problems in this phase of life, all people are psychologically faced with similar challenges. C. G. Jung assumed that the individual fluctuates between his often unconscious true core, the self, and the persona built for contact with others, switching back and forth (cf. Kuehs 2015). The tension between the person someone truly is and the person they present to the outside world can vary in intensity. C. G. Jung distinguishes this concept of self and ego from Freud's conception of the ego, which must defend itself against the demands of the id,

V. Münch, *Group Experience as a Resource*,
https://doi.org/10.1007/978-3-662-70864-4_6

the instinctual side of the personality. Jung rather envisioned a balance between the legitimate demands of the self, which he did not define solely as instinctual, on the one hand, and the ego complex, which is in contact with society, on the other. For many, but especially for narcissistically accented people, midlife represents a threshold situation. For too long, one may have been able to rely on one's "facade", stabilizing one's self-worth with performance and recognition. Fears and avoidance behavior may have solidified, which can lead to people being unable to adequately cope with the psychosocial developmental tasks of the upcoming stages of life. Further rigidity and regression, and thus also illness and premature psychological aging, threaten. In this context, Jung also spoke of the persona, the mask-like, superficial personality, which may be attempted to be maintained, as no alternative experiences and behaviors are available. Psychotherapy or self-experience in general can provide ideas and lead out of dead ends.

The Midlife Crisis and Narcissism

Those who, like narcissistically structured people, are primarily concerned with themselves in a certain way and must regard their own inner world as more significant than that of others, have no sense of the "world" in which other people live, meaning those with fewer narcissistic traits. Such a person also has no idea what others can give them, so that a feeling of being supported and relatedness in a group can be experienced. The diffuse feeling that others can get by without such structural defense arouses strong, unconscious envy in them.

Midlife is the age at which people most often seek therapeutic help due to their difficult psychological development and life's challenges. For many, it is the removal from group contexts and affiliations that contributes to their feeling their life as too burdensome and conflict-ridden. The previous coping strategies, i.e., what has helped to maintain a certain psychological balance, are increasingly failing. No wonder: Either all parameters of success have been reached in external life, or there are increasing signs that certain goals in life are hardly achievable anymore. One reaches a turning point, perhaps feeling at the end of one's tether. Since this is also related to the fact that many people in our Western culture are very much shaped by performance thinking and ideas of eternal fitness, are used to functioning through their everyday life and also the consumerist lifestyle, this can result in an increasingly noticeable inner emptiness. C. G. Jung founded Analytical Psychology itself in such a crisis and contributed the insight that the care of emotional and inner reality can make a more important contribution to satisfaction than the fetishes of our commodity world (cf. Jung 1993).

The Perception of Stagnation in Life

A good portion of my patients, whether female or male, are middle-aged and initially show depression in the face of a stagnating situation at work or in private life. At this point, I would like to focus on an observation that can be discerned again and again in the background of the acute complaints and scenarios. This concerns the fact that many people with problems at this age have few friends, are not integrated into a stable circle of friends, acquaintances, colleagues, or other groups. The circle of friends has become smaller and smaller, people have lost sight of each other (cf. Scharnigg 2023). Others report feeling trapped, caught in a dilemma: Here is the involvement in a job that increasingly dissatisfies them, under- or overburdens them,—there are the increasingly routine family obligations and rituals. One commutes between work and family and is often too exhausted in the evening to find time for marriage or partnership, let alone a personal hobby or the cultivation of friendships, in addition to the obligations. One lives an outwardly "full" life and yet withers inwardly, unable to build real contact anymore. Meetings with friends have become rarer and must always be renegotiated, as there is little regularity in these contacts.

Example

A woman in her late 30s had married early and lived with her older husband and two children. She selflessly cared for the latter, pursued hardly any interests of her own, always striving to be a "perfect mother". Due to her early marriage, she had given up her own professional ambitions early on. In addition to depressive symptoms, she also suffered from psychosomatic complaints. The conflicts with her husband became more intense when she articulated her dissatisfaction. In a long therapy process, the patient developed more self-care and advocated better for her needs. She started making plans more often, toyed with the idea of learning a completely new profession, and redesigned the shared house. Gradually, she was able to lower her high expectations of herself and felt more satisfied. Her marriage was on the brink for a long time, as the husband struggled greatly with his wife's unexpected development and also had to consider changes in his life. In a follow-up conversation years after the treatment, it became clear that the couple had nevertheless managed to stay together. ◄

If you commit a lot to others in the middle of life, take care of them, let yourself be tied up professionally, this is not unusual, as this seems to be laid out by the course of life on the one hand, but on the other hand it is also promoted by prevailing subtle norms in society. Thinking about oneself is quickly considered selfish or narcissistic, the life of the young adult with its playful trying out of new things, the changeable, unstable is considered inappropriate when there is a family to feed and care for. Nevertheless, it is important to create retreats also with people from your own past. Building new circles of friends can also be advisable. It requires spaces where one can be uninhibitedly creative, talkative, musical or sporty-competitive and not only think about one's family or success. This is about truly "free" time, in which one can completely forget about work, as one feels connected with people, ideas, and groups. Phases in which one deals with what used to define one. For many, it is indeed the neglect of hobbies and interests that makes them lose sight of their connection with themselves. The continuity in the life course is lost and with it the former passions and the connection to the guiding inner images. Just like the couples described in Chap. 5, families have a pull: They offer security and safety, they are familiar. On the other hand, when things get difficult or conflict-ridden, the stimuli from outside, the opinions of others, which help to build an internal triangulation to one's own family, a kind of temporarily distanced view, to better recognize and appreciate one's own situation, are missing. Basically, anyone who does not feel that they are still voluntarily involved quickly loses the feeling of inner freedom. Dyadic relationships and also family contexts quickly create the illusion that no other people are needed to be permanently "happy". But it is precisely this permanent happiness that requires these external contacts outside of the dyad or the family. However, there is often too little space for this thought in view of the ideal of the romantic dyadic relationship or the happy family (cf. Illouz 1997).

Slow Regaining of Self-Efficacy

Many patients only begin to slowly, then increasingly, reserve their time for themselves during the course of psychotherapies. Time that was previously often wasted on brooding or dissatisfied lounging on the sofa. The feeling known to most from earlier times, of wanting and being able to actively shape one's own life, returns and enriches the grown relationship. Women in their late 30s often deal with the question of whether they still want to become mothers. Again and again, great pressure arises from unfulfilled wishes, but also in view of the high demands on oneself and potential partners. In therapies, I have often experienced that only when these demands were largely given up and a certain life and self-satisfaction had set in, a pregnancy occurred relatively suddenly and surprisingly.

6.2 Couples Need Groups

While it is true that groups sometimes struggle with couples, it is even more true that couples need contact and integration into groups to function in the long term. It is important that there are separate groups for each partner, as well as groups in which both participate. Shared acquaintances and friends are something that can enliven and stabilize a partnership in the best case scenario. Here, people who care about the happiness of the couple, who can grant the other something without great jealousy because they have arranged their own lives appropriately, are important. On this basis, a creative exchange about shared happiness and about needs and worries can arise, because the shared background is the same at a deeper level for everyone: life and its unexpected twists, the common longing for both security and stability as well as for stimulation and novelty. How important the participation of others in one's own life is and how nourishing and development-promoting it can be, is shown when long-term solitary participants of my groups build a greater openness to changes through the experience and acceptance of their life story and the current life situation: This sometimes leads to someone, contrary to all their own assertions and also the croaking of others, getting to know someone and cautiously starting a partnership. Often these processes are quite unspectacular and quiet, also because the often very vulnerable patients need this protective space. In mid-life, they are usually not so quickly tempted to make gross mistakes, such as wanting to move in together after a few weeks.

Example

A patient who had been in group therapy for a very long period of time found the inner strength to change her life in her own way. After she had extricated herself from an unhappy relationship, she met a "soulmate" with a similarly traumatic life story. Both found the right measure of closeness and distance for them. In the group, she participated more, increasingly making emotional contact with the others. The group eventually became a safe space for her after long phases of fear and mistrust. Her increasing self-acceptance and openness eventually led her to deal once again with her childhood trauma history as a foster child. ◄

6.3 Single and Childless People

Looking at the statistics, many people now live alone, especially in urban areas. A significant proportion of these people living alone are also not in a relationship, are "single" or are looking for a partner. Relatively many of these singles are also childless: In Germany, this currently applies to 29% of all women of childbearing age, almost one in three. Psychologically, in my opinion, it is often the case that people who live alone, and also those who are childless, are less familiar with the experience of the group. This initially circular statement means, however, that these people also think and organize their life and their self-understanding, thus their interpretation of "life" in general, less "group-oriented". Many activities of these people are planned as individual contacts, meetings with couples are less common, probably also because of the feared feelings of jealousy and envy. Naturally, there are often convergences in the topics that concern the participants: Childless couples naturally talk about other topics than their own children and their development. Individual contacts of my single or childless patients are often characterized by exclusivity. Often there are only a few friends or acquaintances with whom there is any contact at all. Sometimes these contacts are also very susceptible to hurt and disappointment, also because they tend to be overloaded with the need to talk and hope for relief. Generally, difficult problem topics dominate rather than simply enjoying free time together.

Overburdening of Partners

On the other hand, some single people also make demands on their partners: that they are open to discussion about their difficult problem topics, their fears and complexes. This is fundamentally okay if it is understood that a couple also communicates and exchanges about their mutual feelings. However, if there is a subliminal elemental desire not to be disappointed, to be fully understood and to have to discuss everything together, then this is often the result of insufficient relationship and bonding experience. Childlike unfulfilled needs are projected onto partnerships. Then relationships can become "pseudo-therapeutic" institutions, especially if the partners initially agree to this and are themselves poor at setting boundaries. This confusion, however, overburdens adult relationships and endangers them (cf. Illouz 1997, 2009, 2016).

Relatively many people are afraid of participating in a group because they tend to find encounters with people rather exhausting. These people are usually parentified, which means that they unconsciously structure their relationships according to the model of their relationship with their parents. Just as they performed a parental function towards their parents as a child, comforting, relieving and guiding them by putting their own needs aside, they often seek people in their lives who also turn to them in their neediness. Some of these patients have almost exclusively problem-laden and exploitative people in their circle of acquaintances. Real friends, i.e., people who accept them as they are and who also listen to them and support them, they have never found. As a result, they fear that this will happen to them again in the group. In the group, the return of the original family constellation is feared, in which one could not defend oneself and resist against abuse and role reversal. Here, psychoanalytically speaking, there is a compulsion to repeat at work, which, according to experience, appears to be more resolvable in groups, as many people are available for triangulation beyond the transference relationship to the therapist.

6.4 Too Much or too Little Loneliness

Many single parents are also overwhelmed with their everyday life. Since they are used to having to cope with almost everything alone, they can eventually no longer imagine that there are support or assistance offers available and that they can really benefit from them. They feel disadvantaged, on the one hand, because the care for the child is limited, and on the other hand, because there may be speculations as to why they did not stay together with the other parent. In groups, they learn how supportive and helpful contacts with other affected people, but also with people in other life contexts, can be.

Example

A former group participant found himself becoming increasingly isolated after the end of his on-off relationship. Over the course of several years, he founded several self-help groups, which, "nomen est omen", eventually became independent and "released" him. This frustrated him greatly, but it became clear to him that it had been a mistake to seek his "happiness" in groups with sometimes very troubled people. Instead, he focused more on his interests and activities and got to know other people who were similarly interested, more active, and happier. ◄

Example

A patient in his 40s had always been very active in groups. He was socially active, played a role as a musician, led groups himself, and liked to work in teams. A few years ago, he had gotten married and now a child had been born. He was constantly torn between his different areas of life and found it difficult to divide his time fairly. He often tended to overburden himself and take on too much. Over the course of a long therapy, he gradually learned to get to know himself better. Whereas before he often "stumbled" into conflict and overload situations and could only understand them in retrospect, he now realized earlier what was emotionally happening within him and was able to steer his actions more appropriately on this basis. ◄

The period in which the much-cited "midlife crisis" (cf. Münch 2016) can arise now extends between approximately the 35th and 50th year of life. The issues are often similar, the developmental tasks that were not tackled often demand a fundamental change from the individual. The fact that this change should be an inner one only becomes clear to some when they have made hasty final decisions. Therefore, in this life situation, it is usually advisable to proceed slowly and with caution. Groups offer the advantage that participants with a "midlife crisis" can engage in lively exchange with others, including older participants. They can thus be supported in being patient with themselves, understanding difficult situations better, and drawing the more sustainable, correct conclusions. As in many other areas, it can be enormously helpful to see and experience that other people are going through similar things. Feeling the resulting connection is part of what can be described as healing. If other people have found solutions, I might also find a solution to my dilemma. One learns to better endure moments of tension and conflicts until a better solution presents itself, a view that is not very popular today in the world of "doers".

Example

For a group participant in his early 50s, his role in his family of origin was repeated in the group: He repeatedly did not get a chance to speak because he himself thought he had nothing important to contribute. He felt lonely here, as often in life, including in his own family. It slowly became clear that he could initially accept very little of the others' compassion in the group. His self-compassion was very weak, ultimately he had a relatively insensitive way of dealing with himself. Only gradually did he let others get close to him. Slowly, a grief over what was missing developed and he found new ways to greater satisfaction, asserting himself more in the professional and domestic context. ◄

References

Illouz, E (1997) Der Konsum der Romantik. Suhrkamp, Frankfurt/M

Illouz, E (2009) Die Errettung der modernen Seele. Suhrkamp, Frankfurt/M

Illouz, E (2016) Warum Liebe weh tut. Suhrkamp, Berlin

Jung, C G (1993) Erinnerungen, Träume, Gedanken. Walter, Düsseldorf

Kuehs, W (2015) C. G. Jungs Definition der Persona und des Selbst. In: Mythenweber. Springer VS, Wiesbaden. https://doi.org/10.1007/978-3-658-09813-1_26

Münch, V (2016) Krise in der Lebensmitte. Springer, Heidelberg

Scharnigg, M (2023) Irgendwann hat man nur noch gute Bekannte. SZ-Online: https://www.sueddeutsche.de/leben/freundschaft-lebenshilfe-maenner-alter-freunde-gute-bekannte-1.5386395?reduced=true#:~:text=M%C3%A4nnerfreundschaftenIrgendwann%20hat%20man%20nur%20noch%20gute%20Bekannte&text=Einsamer%20Wolf%20gut%20und%20sch%C3%B6n,wieder%20mit%20einer%20echten%20Freundschaft%3F

Generativity in Groups

7

Abstract

This chapter deals with the experiences of the "Silver Agers": At the end of their professional lives, most people experience a massive shift in their group affiliations and thus in their group identity. The crucial question is to what extent these changes are experienced as desired and self-determined or as externally determined and abrupt. Here, a variety of adjustment problems can occur.

Example

A patient in his 70s had several partner relationships throughout his life. However, these never lasted more than a few years, so he found himself alone at the threshold of old age. Living alone became increasingly burdensome for him, especially after retiring from his professional life. He suffered from feelings of loneliness and the loss of a "sense of life". He had never pursued his hobbies intensively, and he also found it difficult to fit into groups, such as clubs. ◄

The satisfaction that a communal experience can give has something special. Ultimately, it is the same on a small scale: Shared joy is double joy—whether in a partnership or with friends. The larger the groups become, the more complex the achievements and goals that can be achieved together can be. Many older people appreciate joining a community, for example, singing in a choir. The symbolism of the choir in Greek tragedy was the proclamation of universal truths, and ultimately that is exactly what a choir achieves when it performs classical or religious works. In the large group of a choir, it becomes clear that everyone stands in relation to the whole, but conversely, every individual also matters. If not many others contribute with their characteristic vocal timbre, which represents the whole person,

V. Münch, *Group Experience as a Resource*,
https://doi.org/10.1007/978-3-662-70864-4_7

no overall expression and impression can be achieved. Thus, the individual experiences an unexpected expansion of individual limitations through this possibility of mutual participation in the group "choir". The overall sound of a choir also illustrates well that individuals sometimes become seemingly invisible or inaudible, much like well-integrated participants in a therapeutic group. If you remove the individual voice, the individual participant of a group, the gap is immediately noticeable and the group itself becomes painfully aware of this.

Example

An older patient, who had spent most of her life by her husband's side, suffered from his mood swings. She had given up her own interests, her professional activity, and her relationships largely in favor of her husband and their two children. She became painfully aware late in life that she had put herself in a great dependency. Despite long-term treatment, she found it very difficult to experience and lead her inner and outer life more independently in small steps. She repeatedly fell back into old behaviors and ways of experiencing and seemed desperate in the face of the time that had passed. She found it difficult to let go of the past, as she perceived too little future left. Due to her fragile inner structure, she was afraid to allow strong affects, including grief. ◄

Culture as a Group Achievement

This example makes it very clear that the relationship of the individual to the group and vice versa is very lively, and it is obvious that we humans can only achieve limited constructive things if we work alone. Great tasks of humanity can only be accomplished by many together. Thinking about it, one can only remain in humility and respect in front of the monuments of such community achievements. I think of great architecture, great music in an orchestra, almost every cultural achievement that is only conceivable as a community action.

For many people at the end of their professional life, the question arises as to what contribution they have made to the community, to society. For some, it is a kind of "awakening" after a long time of "functioning" in roles, tasks, and responsibilities. Suddenly, due to the changed societal attributions, one is confronted more with one's own issues, one's own life story, and one's own previous priorities.

Example

After many years of dissatisfaction and overload, a patient in her late 50s took on a new position. This change was apparently only possible after a number of securities had previously collapsed. Illnesses and deaths in her circle of friends confronted her with the finiteness of life, which additionally motivated steps for change. The decision turned out to be very relieving and consistent. More balance and a greater personal sense of freedom were established. ◄

7.1 Early Retirement

About a third of all people, as I recently heard on the radio, receive their pension before the regular retirement age. Numerous forms of early retirement, part-time work for older employees, or other arrangements help people with various physical and especially mental limitations to exit from a work situation they no longer find bearable. This, as we all know, places a great burden on social security systems. Of interest to psychotherapists is the fact that there is a very large number of people who receive this early retirement due to mental limitations, many of whom we should theoretically find in our practices. Unfortunately, this is not too often the case.

As life expectancy in Western industrialized countries has been increasing for a long time, the phase of retirement is getting longer and needs to be financed accordingly. But even more important seems to be that people should start thinking early about what they want to do with the decades they still have available. Many people find a self-determined and active life desirable, but often neglect their own interests during their professional life and alongside their family, so it often comes down to rediscovering these interests and abilities in order to achieve a life in retirement that is perceived as meaningful and satisfying.

Empty-Nest Syndrome

If people have spent their lives, as described in the vignettes mentioned, mostly alone or in a close, traditionally led marriage, they often know less about being involved in groups and the various points of connection that this offers for psychological experience. Groups outside their nuclear family—the family of origin or their own family—have usually played a lesser role. At the latest when their own children move out and become adults, many realize that they may have limited themselves too much to the close family circle. Accordingly, these people experience themselves as being little supported by social contexts. They then perceive themselves as superfluous, as failures, as having been short-changed, sometimes also trapped in a prison of compulsions and dependencies. They receive little support in this, as there are fewer friends and acquaintances, especially those who may have had similar experiences in life and found other ways of coping. Often this also results in the feeling of being overwhelmed, as one feels one has to manage everything alone. However, once a life has been mostly lived, many defense mechanisms have also become entrenched. This makes it harder to bring about and dare to make changes. The painful is at the same time the familiar, in a certain sense even the proven. Any change in behavior, any change in perspective can then cause fear and in turn intensify self-pity and despair, as the past can no longer be changed.

Therefore, treatments of older patients often strongly focus on the development of improved self-acceptance and self-love. This in turn can only succeed if inner freedoms can be conquered beyond the corset of self-reproaches, which is often complained about but familiar. Quite similar to the treatment of narcissistically impaired people, it often involves learning to face the insult that life usually turns out differently than one imagines. The development of humor is essential in this, because those who cannot laugh at themselves find no distance to themselves and their life story. This can be positively influenced much more directly and quickly in group contexts. Paradoxically, in this context, it is about taking oneself less seriously, about a more playful approach to oneself and one's own life, one's own being and having become. Other group participants can become role models here.

7.2 Generativity and the Passing on of Knowledge and Experience

Many people who have always valued contacts outside the family in their lives, people who have nurtured their interests and hobbies, find the transition to retirement less unsettling. They look forward to having more time for themselves and their passions. These can include activities that are mostly done alone, such as gardening, model building or photography, as well as group activities such as hiking, singing in a choir or volunteering for charitable purposes. Also, commitment to a social (marginal) group testifies to the desire to be part of a larger whole, to contribute something meaningful to the common good and to be able to experience exactly that as satisfying (cf. Erikson 1973). Like middle age, which for some perhaps for the first time helps to question the significance of the hitherto prevailing certainties of external and material security, the end of professional life also represents both a danger and an opportunity. The opportunity lies in the reactivation or intensification of connections that can contribute to a life experienced as more fulfilling in social integration. If this does not succeed, the danger lies in a further consolidation of rigid notions of reality and drifting into unrealistic dream worlds and social withdrawal.

Generativity of Groups

Generativity is something that not only individuals, but a group produces. The creative solutions to problems and conflicts that can be achieved through the interaction of several people clearly show that groups have an inherent power and potentiality that can bring forth new things, enable the linking of unfamiliar thoughts, and overall, are capable of elevating emotional processes to a more expressive, differentiated, and communicatively mature level. Groups have emergent properties, they direct the feelings and thoughts of the people coming together in them in a direction they could not have intentionally known beforehand and which often has a surprising quality. Experienced psychotherapists know: What is at the end of a treatment often are not exactly the goals that patients and therapists had in mind at the beginning of the collaboration. Especially in groups, the common search movements and the co-constructive development of the participants as well as their antipathies and sympathies in the course are often unpredictable and can have an immediate effect on the emotional experience of the individuals involved due to this unplanned nature. This can lead to lasting internal structural changes. More on this in Chap. 8.

Focus on One's Own Resources

Consideration must, of course, be given to existing health restrictions. The complaints pointing to one's own transience and limitations can lead to identifying with people who have a more open future. So, when older people engage with younger people and support them, this can strengthen the intergenerational connection.

Social volunteering has a large and socially significant function. People who support school children in their learning or teenagers in their leisure activities, children in learning a sport, bring their lifelong acquired knowledge and ultimately do themselves a favor by reminding themselves in this act of the competencies and skills they possess, what they are still good at. The gift to the younger ones is also a sign of gratitude for what they themselves have received in their life course. And it is an exchange across group boundaries.

In many ways, the image of old age today no longer corresponds to what was understood by it in the past. However, the cheerful and young "old" people propagated by the consumer world are an artificial product if too little attention is paid to the limitations and changed perspectives of the elderly. The elderly are sometimes no longer allowed to be "old", but are forced to deny the more difficult aspects of their lives, which can trigger mental illnesses that were thought to be overcome. Lehofer (2020) has provocatively argued that many of the images we have in our heads about older people are clichés upon closer inspection and that it is more important how older people actually feel internally and emotionally. The perceived age rarely corresponds to the actual age.

Rediscovery and Variation of Previous Interests

Looking back at the dissatisfied people mentioned above, one way would be to lead them back to such an activity that led to satisfaction in the past and thereby reconcile them with themselves at least in part. It is a fine line to consciously shape life, to "celebrate" it in old age, and on the other hand not to make oneself ridiculous. The necessity to recognize limits may mean that leisure activities have to be given up. However, the losses and farewells can be partially compensated by new options. If I can no longer actively practice a sport, I could become a coach or teacher, if I am no longer recognized in my professional field, I can bring its contents closer to laypeople, for example at the adult education center, by explaining the basics of my subject. Or by providing simplified neighborhood assistance, such as an IT person helping older people who are struggling with new communication technology.

When you retire from professional life, it can also feel a bit like the "seriousness of life", which you have been looking forward to since childhood, is supposed to be over, that you are then no longer important to society. Especially those who have defined their identity very much through their profession, even if it may not have been the dream job, are forced to redefine their identity by retirement. In view of the aging society and also against the background of the shortage of skilled workers, the awareness is growing that older people definitely need meaningful and also identity-creating tasks. Many people continue to work on an hourly basis, some because they have to, many because they want to.

7.3 The Age

The group of older people in western countries is growing rapidly. However, many face a lonely and financially restricted old age, as the conditions of life, especially in the big cities, become increasingly adverse and strenuous. Particularly when the life partner is no longer alive, it becomes all the more important to socialize, to join groups. Elderly care facilities support social contacts and the maintenance of interests, wherever possible. But these are changing, as new generations are reaching retirement age, who have led a different life than their own parents. They have different demands on themselves and old age. From a developmental psychology perspective, life means possibilities for change until the end (cf. Schmidbauer 2022). For most older people, this is possible under good medical care, only 18% eventually have to move into a care facility, and only a minority eventually suffer from a form of dementia. The nevertheless often catastrophic portrayal of the situation of the elderly is not exactly encouraging for many. In this regard, a lot of support, orientation, and information is needed. As can be exchanged in a group. These can be interest groups, clubs, offers from social institutions, joint trips, but also self-help groups and therapy groups, depending on the need and necessity.

7.4 Competition and Cooperation

When both the subjective changes in life, such as decreasing physical and mental resilience, physical complaints, as well as the objective signs, such as reaching retirement age, the impossibility of starting an education or being able to take out a loan, show: "The times they are a changing", then aging people find themselves faced with the ambivalently experienced situation of not having to do as much, but at the same time not being able to do as much or even being allowed to. What on the one hand represents a relief, is on the other hand also a "memento mori", announcing further farewells. Younger people tell the older ones that they should now "withdraw from the market", competitions and scholarships of all kinds have an age limit that unmistakably makes it clear: it does not go on here. Quite naturally, however, one suddenly becomes part of the group of pension recipients and has to deal with the fact that some people may still have an image of pensioners as beige windbreaker-wearing and clumsy people.

A Positive Image of Aging

Kruse (2015) describes how a positive image of aging can be built up in oneself. He finds it particularly essential that older people retain the feeling of being needed, of being able to care for others. This strengthens the feeling of being able to remain an important part of society. The contact between generations contained therein is important for both society and individuals in order to be able to age predominantly satisfied. Opportunities for participation and commitment must therefore also be actively created from a political perspective if one does not want to promote divisive tendencies and mental problems in old age. As life continues despite possible restrictions, the question arises as to what alternatives are available. The relationships within family associations usually change, but they do not become less important for people who have become parents and then grandparents. Many are involved in a kind of extended family in clubs or other organizations where people with similar interests come together. The common interests serve as a vehicle to make the actual goal, spending time together, possible. After the "rush hour" of life, many return to their neglected, earlier hobbies and interests. The shared experience comes to the fore again. The energy that the commitment to common projects can give back flows back into individual lives. The experience of being connected remains, if someone has been able to engage in this experience.

Increasing Loneliness in Old Age

There are lonely, older people who certainly maintain contacts, sometimes also in and to groups, but who seem to repeatedly fall back internally into a space where the connection to others and to the world seems to break off. For these people, the departure of the children, also the farewell from professional life is often a difficult step. It is little reflected in society how incisive this phase of life is for many, as it often happens after over 40 years of continuity and reliability of everyday life, which now breaks away. Many people become ill, some do not survive this point for long. However, if today's pensioners were already active and sociable people before their "retirement" (a highly doubtful term), then the chances are good that at least in the pursuit of personal interests a longer continuity awaits them. Otherwise, early deprivations, feelings of loneliness and despair can spread, because there is hardly anything in everyday life that could distract or take up the energy that is now freely available. From psychoanalytic experience, it is often very early experiences in life that can be remembered again in old age or, if experienced as traumatizing, can also occur as "flashbacks". If no help is offered in coping with these experiences, the already fragile defense must again perform a lot, which can lead to hardening and embitterment of the personality.

Group Therapy is the Method of Choice Especially in Old Age

Participation in analytical group psychotherapy can help to alleviate the painfully perceived gap between one's own inner self and other people, to bridge it in the here and now. Often, however, it is about scaling back the still or just once again particularly high expectations of oneself and seeing that one's own glass is half full and not half empty. A benevolent and lenient view of oneself and one's own, sometimes difficult life is hard to achieve if struggling with oneself has already been a lifelong condition. By representing the lively, hopeful, and reconciling own parts, the other group members can offer the opportunity to take back these projections and thus find greater self-acceptance and thereby more inner peace. Overall, psychotherapy is still used too little by older people, measured against the morbidity of this age group and the burdens that have to be shouldered. This requires further education and the commitment of group psychotherapists.

7.5 Living with Transience

Verena Kast (1996) has addressed the topic of transience in many of her books. What is meant is an attitude towards life that appreciates each day against the backdrop of one's own mortality. The attunement to farewells from loved ones and also to our own inevitable departure from life can, in her view, paradoxically help to become a more content and serene person. From the perspective of the bigger picture, everyday troubles become relatively insignificant and we are again more able to gratefully appreciate our resources and strengths. Above all, what connects us with other people can be experienced and enjoyed more intensely, because in this respect all people are truly equal.

The Mourning Community
Even after the end of a life, a group of people usually comes together. Sometimes overwhelmingly many, sometimes only a few. The diversity of people that can be found at a deceased person's grave points to the inner diversity of the deceased person himself, his various tendencies, life worlds and temporal phases in the life course. Representatives of the family origin can be found as well as representatives of an interest-led elective affinity in some cases. Especially people living in big cities root themselves in the most diverse relationships and contexts over the course of their lives. They can benefit from this, provided they remain healthy and mobile, even in old age.

The End of Group-Determined Life
Groups are therefore to be thought of as plural, extended origins. They shape a person on the one hand and reflect his inner diversity on the other. This process is to be thought of as co-constructivist. There is no chicken and no egg, it is difficult to imagine a beginning and a trigger and perhaps this is rather misleading. Groups can bring about balance and correction through their existence, they often work more quietly than explicitly propagating their values. Problems often arise where there is little openness to new groups and thus new influences. The loyalty sometimes paid to the nuclear family can tragically turn against the individual if it is associated with persistence like stagnation and ultimately destruction.

"Anti-Group" would also be effective if even the group itself is avoided, it would be a life against groups—and thus against participation and inclusion, in the truest sense of the word. Participation in something larger is ultimately a spiritual need that can receive some confirmation and response through groups. The turn to faith communities does not have to be explicit. Every group membership is based on a shared system of meaning and a common world of experience. Thus, we find home where we sense commonality, based on the collective dimension of our psyche anchored within us.

References

Lehofer, M (2020) Alter ist eine Illusion. Gräfe und Unzer, München

Erikson, E (1973) Identität und Lebenszyklus. Suhrkamp, Frankfurt/M

Schmidbauer, W (2022) Die großen Fragen des Alterns. Ecowing, Elsbethen

Kast, V (1996) Trauern – Die abschiedliche Existenz. CD. Auditorium Netzwerk, Müllheim

Kruse, A (2015) Wie es gelingt, erfüllt zu altern. Deutschlandfunk: https://www.deutschlandfunkkultur.de/altersforscher-andreas-kruse-wie-es-gelingt-erfuellt-zu-100.html

Part II
Getting Healthy with the Group as a Resource

The Group as a Resource

8

Abstract

The question we want to address in this part of the book concerns the conclusions that can be drawn from the observations in the first part for therapeutic work. What can be worked on? How should work be done? What can be considered effective in analytical group psychotherapies? Many explanations and examples will follow in the next chapters. If it was difficult relationships and group experiences in the past that have had a shaping and inhibiting effect on development, how can new group experiences connect to this, how can the unpleasant experience of repeating traumatic experiences be avoided? And where does the assumption come from that we all carry a need for trustful attachment within us? We want to emphasize the resource orientation in everything, a commonality of Analytical Psychology, contemporary trauma therapy, and modern behavior therapy, as well as, I think, also in the work in groups, as long as their effectiveness is fed by factors that can be particularly effective in groups, but only under certain conditions can unfold. In the end, the conclusion is: Groups work well because our entire lives as humans take place in groups.

8.1 Invitation to Change Perspectives in Psychotherapy

What do I mean when I emphasize how much a group can represent a resource? And what do I mean when I describe that groups are capable of awakening mental resources in the individual, so that conflictual situations can be better managed? In this chapter, we will approach the concepts of Analytical Psychology, which will be further elaborated. It becomes clear that from this perspective, often less needs to be "done" in groups than held and allowed. The task of us therapists is similar to providing a vessel for the developing mental processes.

V. Münch, *Group Experience as a Resource*,
https://doi.org/10.1007/978-3-662-70864-4_8

At every moment in group therapy, the situations mentioned in the Chaps. 3, 4, 5, 6 and 7 from childhood and adolescence are reactivated, especially when the biographical experiences have been unsatisfactory and emotionally burdensome. In addition to the fears of repeating a negative experience, hopes for a good experience are activated. The connection to the mental development that has been halted at certain points can succeed better when the unconscious of the patients themselves takes the lead and the topics and interactions are freely chosen and can take their course as little influenced by the management of the conductors (Foulkes) as possible. Instinctively, those moments of experience that have been missing until then are integrated, either identificatorily as a witness of an interaction between others or "on one's own body" in direct exchange with others including the group conductor. The extent of existing fears determines the speed of the unfolding of the mental landscape and its influence by new, corrective experiences in the group context. Of course, it also happens that the early experiences can be mourned, but only when the secure basis of a new relationship experience is internally anchored.

For Everyone, the Group is a Different Group
From what has been said, it follows that the individually entangled participants, each in a complex way, deal with a different aspect of their emotional situation, such as their self-esteem regulation, at different speeds, while they all apparently deal with the same topic externally. Therefore, one can also say that the group is a different group in the experience of each individual. Only the sum and then the intersection of these different perceptions could offer something like a realistic description of the competencies and characteristics of a specific group.

Example

If we return to that patient who spent a very long time in one of my groups and who was gradually able to deal more calmly with her burdensome fate: For her, the group was presumably that "environmental mother" in the sense of Winnicott or also a transitional space in which new experiences could be made. At the beginning was the experience that the group is perceived as benevolent and accepting. It lets one be as one is, inquiries and insistence are reduced to a minimum in unconscious coordination of the members, in order to first create a trustworthy basis. This is something that as a therapist one does not have to explicitly instruct the group participants, it develops within what unfolds as group ethics or group code, certainly never completely unaffected by the interventions of the leaders. Within this framework, everyone in the group decides for themselves when something is told and when one can and wants to engage in difficult topics. This is the basis for successful work on structure and complexes and conflicts in the future. ◄

The Problem Behavior can be Experienced and Understood Live in the Group

Groups are an underestimated resource in the field of psychotherapy, perhaps because they play such an integral part in all our lives that their fundamental psychological role is not recognized without more thorough consideration. Groups are thus somewhat a kind of "psychological air" that we need to breathe. The concern of those seeking help from psychotherapists is often that they want to have that one person to talk to, with whom they can open up trustingly. However, the help that one can give as a therapist often consists in clarifying the relationships of the individuals concerned, helping them to maintain existing connections, and to seek and establish new contacts. A recommendation for a group can offer these aspects on site and for demonstration. The therapists become witnesses of the observable difficulties to move competently in social contexts. Often, the exact emotional character of the social difficulties is much harder to grasp due to the concealing and contradictory descriptions of patients in individual settings. In the group, completely different countertransference reactions arise, which can then be used beneficially for diagnostics and interventions. Starting from the conflicts that are sometimes very prominently visible in this context, new contacts and new forms of behavior and experience can emerge on a trial basis, which gradually relativize and also help to resolve the previous difficult experiences. Often, over time in a group, it becomes clear why, due to misguided communication, due to a certain impact on others, analytically speaking, due to certain transferences, the relationships of the patients may have been repeatedly disappointing.

What the Group Reveals About the Individuals

The fact that the information that can be obtained in a group context about the behavior of patients often goes far beyond what they know to report in individual settings is partly due to the nature of the unconscious, which, as we know today, consists to a large extent of implicit knowledge, of action knowledge, which in turn does not belong to the dynamically repressed unconscious, but represents a characteristic of humans. Therefore, someone may not be able to give precise information about certain aspects of their experience and behavior, especially in situations of tension and conflict, which are characterized as social situations, because there is (yet) no consciousness about it. Also, usually too strong affects are involved. It is obvious that the information obtained by observing the interactions in the group is very useful therapeutically. The other group members reflect and play in these scenarios always projected parts of the index patients, expressing something that otherwise the close relatives would feel. The understanding for the patients can thus be completed and improved through the many small interactions, through inquiries, comments, emotional reactions overall. In the individual setting, however, a too one-sided representation of others or oneself also becomes noticeable over time. These perceptions, also corresponding countertransference feelings, are however harder to verify. In the therapeutic group, the behavior becomes visible and open for all, which of course can also put pressure on the therapists. The often spontaneous reactions of the other participants can be appropriate, but too early to be processed beneficially by the addressed person. Nevertheless, the process in the group more closely mirrors the real situation in the external life reality of the individuals concerned. A therapeutic group situation, like the dyadic, therapeutic situation, has a partially artificial character—especially due to the unusual rules and framework agreements -, but it contains more features of a "normal" social interaction in non-therapeutic contexts than the individual situation.

Multiple Reflections of One's Own Parts

As a rule, in a so-called slow-open group, i.e., a semi-open, therapeutic group, there are always also members who have been in therapy for a longer time. These, ideally together with the leaders or conductors, create a climate that cushions the spontaneity of others' feedback, so to speak, placing it in the context of the therapeutic process already experienced by themselves. So, in addition to criticism, there is always simultaneous understanding for a described position. The diversity of backgrounds and thus perspectives in a given group allows, on the one hand, that there is always someone who can contribute a roughly similar experience and thus provide understanding and reassurance. On the other hand, there is usually a complementary, supplementary position, which may initially be perceived as "criticism", but is often later recognized by the reporting patients themselves as a projected part of their own personality. Thus, group participants are, on the one hand, under more pressure to communicate than in individual therapy; on the other hand, they are also handled more cautiously, as "a group knows" that things take time. This in turn causes individuals to develop a basic trust in the group as such, in a kind of sensitivity or "group wisdom", which creates trust and encourages further openness.

8.2 The Interaction Between Individuals and Groups

A group thus represents a resource for individuals, as everyone is socialized in groups and knows groups. They are thus referred to potentially desired experiences that were likely disappointed in the past. Hence the great initial fear in some patients. Every single person has internalized negative group experiences, which, it is feared, could be confirmed again. Only slowly does the confidence arise that this group could be a different group, that it, held and protected by the framing therapists, can enable a new experience with others, which can be experienced as relieving, clarifying, and even liberating and connecting. Some patients require a long individual treatment, some find this sufficient. Some need a group experience afterwards, as the individual experience has helped to sufficiently reduce the fear of groups. And some patients, this is probably the most controversial point among group analysts, occasionally need supportive individual conversations even in the group context. Also, to be able to maintain the inner contact to the therapist as a good figure at all. The criticism of this takes the group idea itself into focus and fears an evasion of group dynamics through the use of individual sessions. The arguments that nevertheless speak for the so-called combination therapy are discussed in Sect. 10.6.

The Group is a Resource in the Individual

Theoretically significant is also a thought as formulated in the subheading: Elemental is the assumption that we do not stop at the duality of accustomed thinking and focus on the idea that "the group" has a direct influence on individuals. The group gains its psychological significance for individuals only in that it is experienced as significant intrapsychically. Individuals recognize themselves, so to speak, as always existing parts of groups, as embedded in a network of meaning, communication, and exchange. It is ultimately the psychological resources or resistances of individuals that create "the group", both its existence, its difficulties, and its potential effectiveness. "The group" thus strictly exists only in the individual. The mere gathering of several people for a specific purpose does not yet constitute a group or group experience according to this view. The group experience depends on whether I can internally allow such a gathering of people to be recognized and accepted as a group and as significant for me and my needs. Groups are therefore never effective per se. If the negative pre-experiences are too negative, it can be very difficult to integrate patients into groups and make group participation a positive experience. Here, there can sometimes also be dropouts on the part of the patients or someone may leave the group context to continue working individually.

The Popularity of the Resource Concept

The concept of resource has gained strong momentum in the psychotherapy and self-help landscape over the past one and a half decades. In the context of trauma therapy, it often involves strengthening self-care, regulating self-esteem and affective experiences with the help of "tools", cognitive and behaviorally supported methods that are practiced in self-application and help to better manage unbearable dissociative or panic states and flashbacks. In Analytical Psychology, too, the idea that a large part of the neurotic personality is healthy, that there are always resilient and vital sides of a person, is a foundation. Especially the idea that the unconscious is not merely a repository of the unwanted and repressed, but of vital drives, of the core self, from which the development of the personality unfolds, is deeply convinced of the creative possibilities of humans. What can be criticized is that for a long time little attention was paid to the fact that the individuation of humans is not merely an introverted, solipsistic affair, but always also takes place in the confrontation of the unconscious with the world of others. Here, Analytical Psychology finds its appropriate application within groups.

Example

A male participant in his middle years often appeared very combative and quickly attacked in the group. He also described physical confrontations in his everyday life, quickly got into conflicts. When he was able to recognize with the help of the group that his aggression was understandable from his history with his parents, he felt seen and accepted in these affects. This in turn led to a calming and increased ability for self-control in conflict-ridden situations, also with his parents and siblings. The group had provided a space for the presentation and expression of his anger and had "endured" him. Personal entanglements and complications that resulted from this could be worked on, as there were always other participants who took a more neutral position and helped to deescalate and triangulate. The tendency to escalate could be understood as a desire to be accepted with one's own aggression and not to have to experience it destructively and thus guiltily. Subsequently, the patient devoted himself more to "sublimated" activities such as his creative and musical hobbies and found alternative expression for his personality in them. ◂

8.3 The Group as a Space for Experiencing the Transpersonal, Collective

Connectedness, closeness, and exchange are actually the wrong terms to convey what can be done constructively in a group. They assume that we as individuals must be thought of as psychologically separate and only through exchange and actively induced, reciprocal communication processes such as verbal expressions can we reconnect. Analytical Psychology goes beyond this by assuming that the connections exist unconsciously anyway and that the exchange processes also predominantly take place unconsciously and are not consciously or verbally communicated, yet are effective in their effects as a community experience. An archetypal perspective (see Sect. 14.5.2) also implies that we should include the concept of finality in our understanding of group processes (see Chap. 14). Finality asks, "Where does this want to go?", what developments are inherent in the self of the patients and also in the group self (cf. Vogel 2017)? What wants and can therefore unfold in a group process? As Nitsun (2014) describes, it is precisely the oscillation of a group between constructive and destructive impulses and aspirations that can initiate a creative transformation process of the participants. So a whole series of unfamiliar thoughts for psychoanalysts gather: first the assumption of collective unconscious connectedness, then the hypothesis of a finality, a force influencing the future development of unconscious events, and finally the assumption that the integration of destructive, group-targeted attacks also contributes to the success of the "therapy group" venture. The latter thought is perhaps closest to the familiar hypothesis that the integration of aggression should be a main goal of psychotherapeutic work.

The Group Self

Braun (2016) has explicitly explained how a "group self" unfolds and asserts itself in every psychotherapeutic group over time. This can be understood as an emergent, self-regulating process of unfolding new psychological contents and activating resources, in line with the concept of the self in Analytical Psychology. This group self also has a telos, a finality, of its own. Depending on the individual participants, the personality of the leaders, the theoretical backgrounds and the unconsciously guiding assumptions and the context conditions of the group execution, a group identity is formed, which allows individuals to represent certain values and norms that may not have been a consensus before. Occasionally, as Braun (2016) continues, groups also give themselves designations that are intended to characterize their identity approximately. As is known from social psychology, this process, which can be analytically seen as the identification of the group with its unconscious, represents a stabilization of the group internally and a demarcation externally. This is all the more important given the fundamentally very open initial situation in analytical groups, which brings with it many uncertainties. The new certainties are not reactive defense mechanisms, but creatively refer to the potential of the participants lying ready in the group unconscious.

The Uncontrolled Group Process

In analytical group psychotherapy, there are no specifications about the course and topics. The group embarks on a journey, it is an open process, one looks at what happens. This approach has the advantage that unconscious resistances and fears are also involved in the group process and can thus be integrated into the psychological events. The events constantly oscillate between the increasing involvement of the participants and tendencies to withdraw, between interested openness and silence, between insight, exchange and conflicts between the group participants. Initially, such conflicts are still little fought out, as the cohesion of the group is too weak to be able to control the fears of falling apart or being expelled if one should make oneself unpopular. Gradually, unpleasant aspects of one's own life, then tensions among the participants are addressed. And again and again, parallel to all constructive processes, there is a tendency towards depression, destruction and negativity, which must also be given space (see Sect. 12.2).

The Injured and Restored Sensitivity of the Group Participants

When the vulnerability and fears of the individual participants can increasingly show themselves through the therapeutically provided framework and the growing trust in the developing "group self", the necessity of defense operations decreases, thereby gaining energy, new drive, and motivation for manifest change. This reassurance brings an increased visibility of the sensitivity of all to the fore. Flaßpöhler (2021) has shown that the tension between sensitization and resilience cannot be eliminated. Rather, and this can be demonstrated in successful group processes, an actualization of vulnerability and emotionality paradoxically leads to an increased self-perception and thus also to more self-esteem. As a result, the ability to deal healthily and adequately with problems and demands of everyday life increases. An increased resilience of the individual emerges. Sloterdijk (2009) would also speak of a (social) immunization.

Various, Intertwined Stages of Group Development

The development of individuals in groups largely depends on the capacities of the group. If there are great fears of certain topics and affects among several participants, it will take longer until trust can be built to communicate more consciously about them. Group participants have an unconscious sense of where the resistances, fears, and defenses of the other participants lie and where they can be helpful and useful to them. This can concern the common defense, but also the possibilities to develop. Over time, each group has a common narrative of its history. This includes the positive and negative experiences that were made during the course of group participation, but also the values and goals that, with increasing familiarity, try to bring out the constructive, hopeful, and self-responsible in everyone's life. How slowly these processes proceed and how much uncertainty and fear must be endured can be guessed when, after long periods of apparent standstill, someone "ventures forward" and talks about previously avoided conflicts. Often these are topics such as separation, loss, suppressed anger, and lack of recognition or the needs for being loved or for intimate physicality. The development of both the individual and the group as a whole follows more of an up and down: there are phases of progress and integration, followed by phases of disintegration and fear, sometimes triggered by changes such as new arrivals and farewells in the group.

The experience that there is a non-conscious, non-agreed or unplannable sequence of psychologically effective processes in their group that are beneficially effective can activate hope in patients. This experience, that despite all uncertainty in one's own life and also amidst the often little comprehensible, very layered group process, dynamics are at work that have a constructive, beneficial, promoting influence on the psychological development of those gathered, is an essential factor of therapeutic, here analytical groups. Greater serenity, self-confidence, optimism, and also resilience emerge. Here, the group becomes a place of "good enough mothering" (cf. Winnicott 1960).

Resources Rethought

In academic psychology and work psychology, the terms resources and resilience are often used in a very utilitarian, neoliberal sense of empowering the individual. However, this is not what is meant here. The activation of resources that happens in analytical groups occurs through the partly conscious, but largely unconscious experience of the connectedness of people. It is about not only personally connecting with other people or with one's own strengths, but being able to perceive and experience oneself internally as a "human among humans". The diverse stories of suffering and also positive experiences shared in groups reveal the ubiquity of suffering and the still existing hope in all human life paths. One psychologically integrates oneself into the realm of the all-too-human and thus finds an inner instance capable of providing reassurance, grounding, and confidence. According to the motto: If important other people can share my experiences, then I am no longer alone in the way I perhaps thought before. This connectedness is the result of experiencing resonance and relatedness, which also makes psychotherapies in general positive experience spaces (cf. Jaenicke 2006).

So, the discovery of resources in groups is not primarily about receiving instructions or tips that one then imitates or practices. One is not repeatedly told that one is okay, and then believes it at some point. This would be too simplistic and rarely works given the deeply rooted, negative introjects and beliefs. No, it is more about the underlying assumption in everything said in groups that exchange, reflection, emotional warmth, and confidence are ingredients for something that the psyche needs for its growth. It's not what the other participants say, but *how* they say it and what resonates with it in terms of feelings and experience, that can become effective in me.

Inexhaustibility of Talents and Interests

Finally, others are also those who settle in various forms in the unconscious and shape me. Not to mention the many talents and inclinations of a person that can never be fully lived out and realized in a lifetime. Seen from the side of the unconscious self, the resource of humans par excellence, every person always lives simultaneously in abundance and in the necessity of having to make a selection. Not only the ever-approaching end of life can be a call to us to assemble a somewhat coherent picture of our own life. Things that do not fit well together must also find a place in this picture. This requires a great integration effort, tolerance of ambivalence, and above all humor. People learn to appreciate the proverbial half-full glass of their life and at the same time to bear the half-empty glass more easily. Here too, psychotherapists and other group participants can help by sharing their own perspectives and experiences. The ubiquity of difficulty that can be observed there can make this more acceptable and this leaves behind more reconciled and resilient people.

Less Alone Internally

What groups can achieve is a kind of internal unfolding of the hidden inner group in the individual. It is the realization that one shares aspects of the lives of others without being identical. One is connected, but also separated, but can bear the latter better as a result. The often to be rebuilt experience of the dialectic of opposites, which life sets up through its experiences, makes it possible to create a space in which development can be resumed. Neurotic fixations are often characterized by stuck, one-sided patterns of experience and behavior, by one-sided views of oneself and others and the world. In other words: It is easier to be oneself when one sees that one is not alone with this task, even if it is a different one for each. This process fundamentally moves towards enlivening: The initially burdened, depressive or anxious atmosphere in the group gradually gives way to greater openness and flexibility. This is thanks to the group's container-contained process of working through the transference and the decrease in regression pressure. The development of humor plays a big role in this, which will also be mentioned again later. And one finally also copes better with the unspeakable when one suspects that this belongs to the human condition and is not due to a personal failure. Thus, the discovery of internal disagreement can lead to the experience of the internal group (cf. Kaes 2009) being reflected as an experience of being one among others in a group of individuals and learning to accept oneself in a tension between hope for redemption and fear of failure.

References

Braun, C (2016) Gruppenselbst und Gruppenmatrix. In: Schimkus M, Stuck U (Hrsg.) Selbst, Ich und Wir. Brandes & Apsel Verlag, Frankfurt/M

Flaßpöhler, S (2021) Sensibel. Klett-Cotta, Stuttgart

Jaenicke, C (2006) Das Risiko der Verbundenheit. Klett-Cotta, Stuttgart

Kaes, R (2009) Innere Gruppen und psychische Gruppalität: Entstehung und Hintergründe eines Konzepts. Psyche 63C (3): 281–305

Nitsun, M (2014) The Anti-Group. Routledge, London

Sloterdijk, P (2009) Du musst dein Leben ändern. Suhrkamp, Frankfurt

Winnicott, D W (1960) The theory of the parent-infant relationship. International Journal of Psychoanalysis, 41: 585–595

Vogel, R T (2017) Individuation und Wandlung. Kohlhammer, Stuttgart

9 Self-Experience Groups

Abstract

In the first part, we discussed a lot about natural group formations. Groups that arise from familial backgrounds, groups that emerge from common interests. In addition to explicit therapy groups, there are many groups in which people want to get to know themselves better, want to develop themselves, want to familiarize themselves with their own possibilities and limitations. Therefore, these groups will be briefly introduced here. The advantages and disadvantages of their structure should be clarified, differences to therapeutic groups should be highlighted.

9.1 A Broad Definition of the Concept of Self-Experience

Beyond the services offered by statutory psychotherapists, who conduct analytical, depth psychological, behavioral or systemic individual and group psychotherapy, there is a variety of contentually and qualitatively very different offers for self-experience also in groups on the "market" for life assistance and self-experience. With the Encounter movement of the 1960s, a whole range of offers have developed, especially in the area of body-related and meditative practices, which are sometimes, but not always, led by trained psychologists. I am thinking, for example, of groups that offer sweat lodge experiences, based on shamanic practices, of groups that deal with breathing techniques such as holotropic breathing or elements from Tantra Yoga. For men and women, a larger market of gender-separated groups has emerged, which have the most diverse thematic focuses. Often it is about exchanging and strengthening each other and helping to reduce the often great dependence on partners. Sometimes the mythological area is extensively used to structure the contents of the group experiences. The seminars or weekends

V. Münch, *Group Experience as a Resource*,
https://doi.org/10.1007/978-3-662-70864-4_9

are then called "the healer", "the warrior", "the king" or "the lover" and deal here with the different dimensions of being a man. An example were the courses by Peter A. Schröter (2012). In terms of content, rituals and exercises are often carried out, often also as partner exercises, in which the experience of one's own body, one's own emotions are in the foreground, without these being extensively discussed in relation to their connection to the biography or to the relationships outside the seminars. In this context, although often intense emotion-based experiences are created, these can often only be shared within the circle of participants and therefore often lose their effect and sustainability after the end of the meetings. Some participants are then motivated by this phenomenon to sign up for the next seminar, which can lead to a new development of dependency, which in turn usually remains unreflected.

Example

A young man who grew up with his mother without his father initially seemed very trapped within himself, trying to solve all problems with consideration. He suffered from panic attacks. I noticed that he found a very pictorial expression for his inner conflicts in the unconscious, in his dreams, but initially could not understand these images as a part of himself, let alone in terms of content. At some point during his long individual treatment, he completed a "men's weekend" and was able to give a differentiated report about what he liked and what he found problematic. The direct experience with other men inspired him to start martial arts training and make new experiences with himself and his body and self-experience. He had clarifying, albeit disappointing conversations for him with his father. Gradually, he was able to stabilize himself overall, soon lived in a stable partnership. ◀

Group Experiences in Theme-Centered Groups During Individual Therapy

As described above, I have occasionally had the experience that some clients were able to have a good, helpful and triangulating experience in such courses. They developed a more differentiated view of themselves, as they were able to share and also expand, check and possibly relativize their previous therapy experience with other participants and another therapist or leader. As an individual therapist who knows about the potency of groups, I do not prevent patients from participating in such groups, as long as they appear serious to me and the patients have become securely attached and also more psychologically resilient in the therapeutic relationship. The discussions about the experiences made there can greatly enrich the individual therapy, similar to the experiences made in the therapy group with me, which also mean a change of perspective for the patients. The multiperspective picture that they receive from the treating person from the beginning promotes their development and limits regression. In this respect, the setting of the so-called combination therapy (cf. Sect. 10.6) is ideal for patients with structural deficits and also for those with mild traumatic experiences such as a cumulative attachment or relationship trauma.

If the seminars are led by trained psychotherapists who are also approved, one can be reasonably sure that regressive processes, which sometimes occur in such group events, are well caught. Personal experiences with courses and leaders are helpful. If one is skeptical, it is better to listen to the inner voice and examine with the patients why they want to go there right now. This examination is of course independent of this, it is about understanding what is being sought outside the dyadic situation. Often enough, the search movements are contentually and emotionally well comprehensible and founded in the history of the patients. Therefore, it is not about prohibitions or taboos, but about a prejudice-free examination of the emerging curiosity and exploration behavior. Only then can the defensive character also be understood together.

Dangers and Opportunities of Alternative Body-Oriented Therapies
Analytical psychotherapy in particular offers so much profound knowledge that there is no need to hastily look at other competitors with jealousy or disdain. Analytical knowledge helps to appropriately assess and evaluate the content and forms of formats offered on the "free market" of group self-experience. A critical but also tolerant approach to many methods, such as those originating from the field of humanistic therapy forms, is helpful. These include, for example, concentrative movement therapy, Gestalt therapy, relaxation methods, body-oriented methods, and meditation practices. But also less serious methods such as the men's group at Pro Familia or the body therapeutic annual group in bioenergetic analysis, the yoga group, and the initiation rituals of indigenous origin shaped by archetypal content can be subjectively perceived as helpful—there is a wide variety of offers both within and outside the so-called esoteric scene. They find interest among some patients, often suffering from structural problems. A certain quality criterion for such self-experience opportunities is certainly a high-quality training of the conductors. And again, good group experiences of the participants. Groups exert a relatively large, regressive pull. Especially in unpredictable, open-ended and surprising seminars, where the participants are supposed to be confronted with their fears, it is important that the groups also fulfill a supportive function. The experience of the individual that others can witness my experience in my presence, as well as I participate in the experiences of others, creates connections on a more elemental level. Here, spaces are pre-shaped to be able to have certain experiences. These can be impressive for the individual participants, but in the long term they often cannot become structurally effective, as too little contact can be made with the real other, with the other participants, as everyone finally separates after days. This ultimately does not achieve the internalization of a relationship experience that has a changing effect. Often, the group dynamic processes when transitioning from the small group to the large group dynamics are not sufficiently considered and psychologically unstable participants are then left alone with their fears!

In a continuous analytical group, however, the participants gradually get to know each other better and deeper, which then leads to sustainable changes through identification, the experience of empathy of others, confrontation, improved perception of one's own feelings and also improved communication of the same.

Knowledge of Alternative Methods

A good knowledge of alternative methods, their dangers as well as opportunities, is helpful for psychotherapists, as it is not uncommon for patients to inform themselves about such methods and also book them parallel to psychotherapy. In this case, it is better if the treating persons show some interest, so that the parallel self-experience is not completed in secret. In this case, the experiences made there are also not usable and integrable for psychotherapy. It also seems important in connection with body-related approaches to know which emotional processes are to be expected with which sports, movement teachings and meditation practices. Especially intensive practices, such as those associated with breath work, are rather critically evaluated, especially for patients with little structure. In this case, participation should also be explicitly discouraged!

Example

A group participant, from whom I had not heard for a long time, contacted me again. In our "crisis talk", which consisted more of her telling me her further life story, it became clear that she had benefited from the analytical therapy. In her eyes, however, she had even developed extremely positively, had dealt with many body-related and generally considered esoteric methods. She had trained in some methods and ran a practice as a naturopath on this basis. She seemed extremely satisfied and at peace with herself, yet I had to think that she had obviously completely identified with her ego ideal. I saw that she therefore no longer showed any suffering pressure and also no further willingness to undergo treatment. ◄

9.2 Milieu Therapy

The form of group psychotherapy, primarily used in a clinical setting, brought to Germany by the psychiatrist Günter Ammon, has been particularly perpetuated within the DAP (German Academy for Psychoanalysis). This is referred to as "milieu therapy" when patients are given project-related common tasks within group-analytical settings. The dynamics that unfold during the joint activity in the small group are regularly discussed in group sessions. In addition, the small groups come together in large group sessions with other groups. The participants are thus also shown that everyone has constructive contributions that are important for the group and the success of a project and can contribute these. This group concept from the treatment of more severe mental disorders already has a modern resource orientation. The concept was conceptualized in the course of the "dynamic psychiatry" movement of the American psychoanalyst Menninger. Ammon, along with others, founded his own clinic in Munich, which still exists today (Klinik Menterschwaige) (https://www.klinik-menterschwaige.de/home/geschichte). This setting has proven to be very effective, especially for very chronic patients who require a long duration of treatment.

9.3 Self-Help Groups

The promotion of self-help groups in the psychosocial field, which is mainly due to Michael-Lukas Moeller in the German-speaking world, should not be underestimated. In a wide variety of groups, those affected find nationwide support from other affected people who have trained to become group leaders. Self-help groups do not see themselves as therapy, there are no leaders in the sense that topics are predetermined. Only the structure and framework should be provided and maintained by the person in charge. Moeller was also concerned with helping people affected by mental problems discover and creatively use their resources. Recognizing the potential of groups, he laid down his thoughts 1978 in his book *Self-Help Groups*. Beyond this, Moeller has given a lot of profound thought to group and pair dynamics against a systemic-psychoanalytic background. Self-help groups today represent an important pillar of the psychological care of the population in Germany. Especially patients with more severe, chronic disorders often participate for many years. The conductors of these groups are, as mentioned, mostly themselves predominantly recovered sufferers. They often show an intense interest in the design of the groups and also in further education and supervision by psychotherapeutic professionals.

Alcoholics Anonymous and Co.

Self-help groups are widely spread in the field of addiction prevention and treatment. Even though the sometimes quasi-religious character and the very superego-heavy structure of some associations are viewed more critically today, these groups are often a great support for those severely affected. One can criticize that in this way, without a causal treatment in the depth-psychological sense, a very damaging dependency is often replaced by a new, less damaging one. Internal, structural changes are less achievable in this way.

References

Moeller, M L (1978) Selbsthilfegruppen. Rowohlt, Reinbek

Schröter, P (2012) Die Kraft der männlichen Sexualität – Lebensbilder für Männer. Piper, München

Therapy Groups

10

Abstract

How does a therapy group work and what are the key components of successful group psychotherapeutic work? Which patients benefit most from groups? How and when should individual and group therapy be used together? What conflicts and difficulties can arise from this? These questions will be addressed in depth in this chapter. We will first deal with the differences and dividing lines, but also the similarities between individual and group therapy.

10.1 Individual and Group Therapy

Patients are always initially seen in a one-on-one consultation in the practice. From this familiar situation, it is often not easy to motivate patients to participate in group therapy. Quite a few people are skeptical and fearful that they will not be able to have the therapists "for themselves" alone, that they may not be able to open up as much as they think they should out of fear. Past experiences from groups such as the family of origin are formative and have often left deep wounds that have buried the hope of a positive, healing experience in groups. This is understandable and requires a lot of tact from the therapists: On the one hand, it is about accepting these fears and making them more understandable to the patients, on the other hand, they must be able to credibly convey from their own experience that and how groups can work. Under no circumstances should the impression arise that patients are being "pushed" into a group because individual treatment is considered too difficult. On the contrary, there needs to be a notion in the therapist that participation in a group is a plus, a gift to the individual patients and also the existing participants, which I am not able to offer in individual therapy. The multitude of group members, their different life backgrounds, the different experiences

V. Münch, *Group Experience as a Resource*,
https://doi.org/10.1007/978-3-662-70864-4_10

and the resulting multiple perspectives can initiate a profound, complex process of identifications, which ultimately leads to more integration. Here I am confronted with my limitations as an individual therapist, I must therefore acknowledge them! I personally know a number of analytical group therapists who lead several groups each week, many do so with increasing enthusiasm and motivation. Due to the then existing different composition and characteristics of the individual groups, new patients can also be more specifically assigned to the groups that "fit" them.

Corrective emotional experiences in group psychotherapy

Belief in the added value of the group thus also includes the insight that patients in the group can make new experiences in "real time" that are often so difficult for them to make in their external life reality. This is because the projections that otherwise lead to constantly repeating, frustrating experiences can be better caught and understood in a therapy group. At the same time, participation in the group also counteracts the narcissistically tinged view that the experiences gained in the individual setting alone lead to a changed self-perception and also perception of others. The latter is particularly the case when the real external relationships and their internal representations find too little entry into the therapy. Ultimately, all therapists always deal with images, with narratives, with interpretations of the psyche about the "others". Psychoanalysts have good concepts for this that are able to depict this. They speak of "inner objects", of representations. Nevertheless, there is also a real level of relationships, which, however, becomes too little clear in individual therapies. I cannot observe the behavior of patients in their everyday life. It is often very revealing when patients are seen behaving so differently towards others in their real behavior and in group behavior after individual treatment or during a parallel individual treatment as part of a combination therapy individual-group. It is clear that this is also influenced by transfer readiness. How difficult some of them find it in groups then becomes overly clear and the individual processes that lead to this can only be examined more closely when the perceptions of the group participants about a patient are considered in an overall view and conclusions can be drawn from this about the repressed parts in the psyche of the person concerned. Here, the deepest conflicts can become overly clear as if under a magnifying glass.

Better overview of external transferences

Group therapy can also effectively address another malaise of individual therapy: it can thus give less false progress. I am referring to the unfortunate situation where a patient shows significant opening and integration in the individual setting, but the external environment of his relationships at home counteracts and often destroys all efforts. This sometimes leads to escalation and separation, in the private environment or also within the therapeutic relationship, where perhaps an understanding would still have been possible. Individual therapy can thus lead to the misunderstanding that the strengthening and stabilization of patients, their empowerment for more self-care and enforcement "against" others and their needs is directed. Since in reality there is often unconscious dependence also because there are needs for unconscious dependence, this layer remains largely unnoticed. That it is always about a changed, new togetherness with the familiar social contacts becomes visible and tangible more quickly in a group. Group participants are generally good in their feedback and comments at striking a balance between the different aspirations perceived in the "index patient". This makes some, even unwanted and premature decisions less likely.

Demarcation as an apparent panacea
The emphasis on the pole of autonomy in treatments has a very real side and a culturally historical aspect: The emancipation movement of the 1960s also massively promoted the belief in the importance of liberating the subject from societal constraints in the field of psychotherapy. This, of course, has its justification when it comes to rebellion against confinement, patronization, and oppression. The drawing of boundaries, or "demarcation," as the first step in therapy and as a now common everyday term, is a milestone in the formation of the subject. By directing attention to this aspect of human relationships, much suffering has already been alleviated. However, it must be noted that this has also given society and the groups within it a predominantly bad reputation, which they are still struggling with today. The one-sided fixation on autonomy, self-realization, and independence now leads to paradoxical developments, such as in the search for a partner (cf. Illouz 2016).

The fact that life is always a coexistence that also requires compromises, which could not only be experienced as renunciation but also as enrichment, is an insight that currently finds too few supporters. The fact that groups always offer added value that exceeds the sum of the knowledge of their participants is even less common knowledge. Ego-centrism in our culture has not stopped at therapeutic schools and expectations of them. The "I" and "we," the subject and its social integration, can hardly be thought of together, and the contribution of the group to the development of the individual is systematically underestimated, also, as described elsewhere, because development is often merely thought of as something that occurs *within* the individual.

10.1.1 Group Aspects in Individual Treatment

What perspective of group therapists can enrich the individual session and what questions arise in this regard? Especially in long therapies, one should repeatedly deal with whether patients are able or willing to implement the insights and progress gained in the sessions in "real" life outside of therapy. Some, especially severely depressive and self-uncertain and also particularly narcissistic or schizoid patients, find this particularly difficult. If one gets the impression that the relationships of the patients do not really change, if difficult relationships with acquaintances and friends continue unchanged, if new, pleasing, enriching contacts hardly ever come about, then one should investigate. From the first part of this book, it should have become clear that the biographical anamnesis should focus on the "group history" of the individual in addition to dyadic relationships. This is not only important with regard to suitability for a possible later group participation, but generally a statement about how much space the group idea plays in a person's life, how integrated he "stands in the world," how much he is able to share the "facts of life" in the sense of Money-Kyrle (1971). Because the limitations of human life are obviously easier to bear when they can be experienced and communicated together. The entire cultural production of humanity, which largely represents a group phenomenon, is shaped by these themes and the countless variants of their representation.

10.2 Group Capability

In order to be able to experience participation in group psychotherapy as helpful, a certain ego strength is required. If I am reasonably sure about my position in reality, about my values and feelings, then I can mentally delimit myself from initially foreign others in order to maintain this existing ego feeling. At the same time, however, I am only then sure enough to be able to take another step towards the others. Curiosity about the experiences of others, the partial ability to change perspective, even empathy for others is difficult if I have not yet had these experiences myself and therefore everything in my world has to revolve around me psychologically. If there is so little identity and ego stability in dealing with reality, every contact represents a danger. I could be confronted with my own inner lack of opinion and placelessness, which can trigger great fear of self-loss.

Preparation for the Group in an Individual Setting

The suggestion to such patients to be able to participate in a group can therefore cause great fear. It is always sensible to offer a certain number of supportive individual sessions before group participation can be considered. Good preparation is required, the fears must be addressed and examined. Occasionally, this phase of therapy may extend over half a year. The innovation of combination therapy also allows this arrangement. The already existing group participants are introduced in individual conversations, the group process and the group rules are described exemplarily. This can reduce fears. The relationship with the therapists deepens over time. Only when the therapists are perceived as a safe object can it be dared to confront a multitude of "others" in the presence of this object. The term "group capability" is very vague from a professional point of view, but is usually intended to describe the risk of malignant regression. Patients who tend to regress and fear due to their fragile mental structure could then react with strong defense, usually aggression, devaluation, and contact breaks. We will describe this problem in more detail in the chapter on narcissistic disorders in the group context (Sect. 11.1). Of course, this is not a size that can be determined absolutely. Much always depends on the therapeutic relationship between patient and conductor. In any case, a lot of clarification work is required for both the group and the patients in this constellation. This means that the difficulties of the new patients are explained to the group as well as the functioning and processes in the group are explained to the problematic patients.

Example

A woman in her mid-thirties, who had always made herself very dependent on others in relationships and at work due to her neediness and was often exploited, initially expressed great skepticism towards the group. When she came into the group after some time, it quickly became apparent that she received from different participants what she had previously hoped for in the dyadic relationship with me: attention, interest, goodwill. The appreciation of others for her own contributions also led to her developing more self-strength and independence over time and the previously conflictual staging of her own neediness with simultaneous resentment due to the perceived inferiority significantly receded. Her depressive symptoms also receded in parallel. ◄

The Schopenhauer Cure

Irvin Yalom's novel character Philip, a strongly narcissistically accented personality, is admitted to a therapy group in the novel *The Schopenhauer Cure* by Yalom's alter ego, Julius, despite considerable doubts. Yalom has Julius convey the realization that the very first acquaintance in a new group is usually much less unpleasant and emotionally difficult than most fear in their imagination (cf. Yalom 2005). Due to the initially large projections that are made due to the lack of concrete experiences, a rather pleasant real experience occurs.

Group capability could also be described as the ability of a group to deal appropriately with new members from a change of perspective. A multitude of adjustment processes take place when a new member joins the group. A group that has been together for a long time has enough sensitivity to greet new members cautiously. The group senses the fears that exist in the newcomer and usually only asks as much as necessary at the beginning. It leaves enough room to orientate oneself in the group and initially make some "model learning" possible. This works once again via the often mentioned, immanent and rarely verbalized aspects of group work. A new member is not endlessly lectured and enlightened "how it works here", but the group creates and offers the opportunity to listen and watch, to be able to see how the interaction and values in the group are determined. If the group process can unfold freely, then relationship disorders and transferences show up here and now. However, they are usually not interpreted so soon, but others in the group react directly to them. This distinguishes the analytical group strongly from the classic analysis, somewhat less from a dialogically oriented, intersubjective relationship design in the analysis. For Yalom, it is also about "interpersonal learning". The clarification brought about leads to a new experience and thus to intra- and interpersonal psychological change (cf. Arndt, Peer et al.: 2011. Psychosomatics and Psychotherapy, p. 150).

10.3 The Influence of Individual Therapeutic Thinking

Another problem often only becomes apparent in group analytical practice: In the application of group therapeutic concepts, many therapists occasionally revert to individual analytical concepts, not always utilizing the potential that can lie in group interpretations. Dalal (1998) in particular criticizes that Foulkes, in his application examples, too often tried to apply classical psychoanalytic ideas, even though he had previously identified the limitations of their applicability for group analysis. Perhaps this is due to the special demands on the leaders or conductors of psychotherapeutic groups. Groups are complex and multifaceted and psychologically significant at various levels. In addition to the real level of adult individuals who want to deal with their problems, there is initially the level of transference of old relationship patterns that want to be reenacted. Depending on the composition of the group and the self-claim of the conductor, group sessions can sometimes be experienced as very strenuous. As a therapist, I also get into a pull, a regressive experience, when it comes to topics that concern early, poorly definable content. To put it pointedly, it can happen that the conductors in a group can fall for an anti-group dynamic (see Sect. 12.2), namely when they cannot grant the group creative solutions, no potential for change, have too little trust in the group itself and therefore try to control everything themselves by interpreting quickly and a lot. This is usually answered by the group participants with counter-developments, setbacks and sometimes subtle aggressions.

In summary and simplified, one could say that interpretations that concern the personal, biographically anchored psychodynamics represent an "individual work in front of the group" and less characterize a work that is related to the group as a whole, interpreting, understanding work. If I have a group in front of me, I should abandon my individual therapeutic attitude for the benefit of the group.

10.3.1 Demarcation and Individuation

As already hinted at above, various newer findings from psychotherapeutic practice and theory suggest that we have probably thought of individuation too individualistically or better too narcissistically so far. The ideas that shape our culture about how autonomy should be achieved and what it should include have also not stopped at the therapeutic schools in a certain way. Not surprising, but one may ask how one should appropriately respond to a misunderstood idea of self-realization in many patients. And this applies to both psychoanalysis and analytical psychology! The main theme in the initial phase of the majority of psychotherapies is, in my experience, the desire for increased demarcation ability. One wants to learn to say no, one wants to "find oneself more", "listen more to one's own voice". This is never wrong, but it is difficult to recognize this as the highest motto, since the needs of others can be just as legitimate and our patients want to feel needed by these other people at the same time. Sometimes the self-perception as submissive and reserved does not match the manifest behavior towards the treating person at all! An individual approach is always necessary, which requires great sensitivity here. When it comes to therapy goals, it should soon become clear that individuation always also means development towards other people. Demarcation always happens *in* contact with others and can succeed more securely and calmly if one can be sure of the enduring connection with others.

Saying no in the group as an important act of demarcation is expressly desired. The no to the group must be questioned more thoroughly.

10.4 Differences Single Analysis—Group Analysis: The Group Interprets

C. G. Jung well described that psychological development is something that not only relates to the individual and depends on his resistances and defenses, by assuming that the psyche is something we are entwined in. He spoke of the "objective psyche" as the part where the not self-acquired, but innate, collective parts of the psyche are located (cf. Jung 1995). In his psychology, the psyche cannot be seen as something that occurs "in the head" of the person concerned, a view that seemed to be supported by the findings of brain research. The psyche is everywhere and we participate in it. This also indirectly always refers to the group idea, although this was not intended by Jung. Giegerich (2012) has very extensively and differentiatedly brought this knowledge to light. At the core, it is about overestimating what we can know when we talk about the unconscious and the soul. Too quickly, we in the psychoanalytic profession tend to talk about insights into the unconscious, that the unconscious has become conscious. If you look at the results of treatments, this fact seems to be given the least importance. The changes that patients report are rather those that suggest a changed inner positioning, a grown ability to trust in oneself and to let one's own decisions be guided more by this newly or rediscovered inner voice. It is rather unpleasant for those people who are able to report on many insights into their psychological mechanisms, but in whose actual external life sometimes very little change or development takes place. This makes a Jungian-influenced analyst think that the changes that are experienced through groups and in groups often rely on participation in archetypal factors such as the experience of belonging. Apparently, what is understood as insight is sometimes interpreted too one-sidedly. The British group psychoanalyst Dalal (1998) has impressively described how group-specific factors beyond "insight" can be decisive for change processes. Heinz Kohut's "How Does Psychoanalysis Cure" (1989) is also critical of the classical analytical view.

Opening of the Individual Setting and the Group Setting to Variations

Against this background, it seems sensible to consider the behavior of a group as a whole, similar to in individual analysis, and to always understand disturbances (by individuals) as a symptom of the unconscious events in the group. There are colleagues who hold the position that the framework of the group should be considered essential, which would have consequences for the feasibility of parallel individual work ("combination therapy"). There are arguments for this, but in my opinion, they go back to a relatively narrowly led concept of transference. In my experience, transference and resistance also unfold in the setting of a combination therapy, even if they can become more complicated. Similar to the discussion about the intersubjective turn in psychoanalysis, in my opinion, it is still too little recognized that part of the professional therapeutic relationship always also is the real relationship, the dialogical, adult side of the relationship, that has an influence on the complex therapeutic relationship and also on the healing process. As we know from the discussion about the "now-moments" (cf. Stern 2018), interventions outside the framework sometimes provide a decisive impulse for changes in treatments. I am explicitly not talking about rule violations and assaults! Rather, I have in mind the complicated reality of various patients with different prerequisites for group psychotherapy or analysis, to which I as a therapist also react differently. Neutrality in the sense of equal reactions to all seems to me to be a hardly achievable demand. This, however, is about the "containing" of the conductor, his ability to endure unspoken, even unconscious aspects of the events and to hold and gradually "metabolize" them. Gradually, the group takes over this function when a development process gets underway. Of course, the personality, experiences with groups, transferences, demands on their work of analysts also play a role. Lesmeister (2017) has subjected this desire of the analyst to a critical analysis.

10.5 Combination Therapy

Finally, let's come to the contentious point of discussion in today's group analysis and therapy: the possibility of combination therapy. For several years now, in guideline psychotherapy in Germany, there has been the possibility to offer group therapy and individual therapy together and to bill them in parallel. Recently, even depth psychology-based and analytical psychotherapy can be combined. In a scope adapted to the individual case, individual sessions are conducted in addition to the continuous, usually weekly group, mostly for support when the patients do not have enough structural prerequisites to benefit sufficiently from the group. If, for example, the tendency to project is too great due to illness, a group is quickly perceived as threatening and hostile, or at least very foreign. The therapists then take on the role of supporters and mediators. The triangulating space between the settings can promote development. The therapist is experienced differently in the different settings, which facilitates the acceptance of the different "sides" of the therapist and thus also increases the inner flexibility and frustration tolerance of the patient. The more differentiated and comprehensive picture of the therapist also brings more divergent aspects of one's own personality into focus. Excessive, defensive idealization in individual therapy is also countered in this way. The therapy setting of combination therapy also has the advantage that it better reflects reality. We are all always alone and involved in (several) groups at the same time. Sometimes it's just about us, sometimes it's about finding our place among others and in the world. And these two aspects can thus be considered and understood together, especially in their difference and interaction.

10.6 Dyadic and Triangulated Relationships in Combination Treatment

Group therapists who have committed themselves to the ideas, theories, and practice of group therapy or analysis, as already touched upon above, sometimes find it difficult to engage in combination treatment. By granting individual sessions differently, we create different conditions for the participants, they say, and we dilute the methodology and what analytical group therapy can achieve. In addition, the unconscious of the group may possibly change. I would counter that the unconscious of the group is certainly changed by this, but it is then more a mirror of the social external reality. I would rather see this as an opportunity than a risk. If different participants in a group receive individual sessions at different frequencies, *can* this generate envy and resentment. However, if this situation is openly negotiated, then this difference can also be better tolerated. The artificial situation of individual analysis with a sometimes misunderstood abstinence and the purity idea of an undisturbed unfolding of the transference, which in my opinion comes from the scientific ideal of psychoanalysis, is transferred by some to groups. By trying to eliminate disturbance variables, which can never be excluded, and by also trying to create an artificial situation compared to the actual real life conditions, one commits oneself to a high ideal.

Certainly, regression is limited when the interactive and social behavior is put in the center. In my experience, however, the new experiences in these dimensions have an impact on intrapsychic structures such as frustration tolerance, psychological resilience, attachment ability, and the ability to humor. In the end, with parallel individual and group work, both a too great fear of symbiosis in the individual setting, but also in the case that the group as a whole is perceived as potentially engulfing, can be successfully triangulated. This does not deny fears, but provides a development-promoting and supportive environment that helps patients to find their way out of their inner entanglements through alternative experience formation. Often it is then only possible to recognize and name the previous arrests and neurotic fixations more precisely in retrospect and also biographically. This also facilitates the detachment from introjected objects and has a positive influence on the formation of internal structure.

Group Therapy as an Experience of the Social Constitution of the Self

The different life paths and personality structures and the resulting differences are always present in groups. They also require different treatment paths. There is no methodology that can be right for everyone, not even with the same disorder. In practice, this means that I also react differently in group therapies to all participants, depending on the internal conditions and individual psychodynamics. If I want to work from the consideration of technical "purity" or from the claim that group therapy, as it exists today, represents the end of development, I am trapped in a construct. Something similar would be the previous attitude of therapists that no life-important decisions should be made during an analysis. This admonition makes sense, as one should be aware of one's regression. Nevertheless, any kind of therapy always represents only a section in the life of the individual. And the therapeutic methods, including the analytical one, continue to evolve! For the individual participants, there are areas of life that exist relatively unscathed alongside neurotic compromises, areas of life that can certainly be considered healthy. Often it is rather a symptom than a truth when patients only see problems in their life and their healthy parts receive far too little weight. Here, group therapy can straighten out a lot and strengthen the healthy parts and thus help weaken the neurotic ones. It is precisely this corrective experience that can significantly contribute to therapy successes in groups.

How many individual therapy paths, how many creative combination possibilities in therapeutic practice today are usable, is shown by the work of Türk (2020). Especially with the often structurally more severely impaired patients, the possibilities of combination treatment are usable and are apparently now also being used more frequently. It is diagnostically very revealing to study how differently patients behave in individual contact and in group context and also how they experience themselves there. Especially at the interfaces of the observable difference in experience and behavior, also in countertransference, a lot of diagnostically and therapeutically usable material can be brought to light. The reactions to the different demands from this therapeutic reality can be observed, accompanied, and understood together.

10.7 Difficult Cases: When Individual Therapy is Not Enough

As a simultaneous individual and group analyst, one sometimes experiences that certain patients, especially those with more severe narcissistic pathologies, are quickly and often for a long time engaged in a defensive struggle against too much closeness and the feared overwhelming in the therapeutic dyad. When such patients come into a group, one sees how difficult they find it to make genuine contact with others, and one gets an even clearer sense of the tragedy of their social lives. Many of them systematically make themselves unpopular with abstract, often self-deprecating statements, with which they want to preempt criticism. Their need for control is overwhelming, probably the transmission of traumatic personal experiences of being overwhelmed by their caregivers. Their statements quickly seem remote from life, they do not really tell about their everyday life, because nothing they fear as much as arriving in mediocrity, which they like to attribute to others. Accordingly, they radiate arrogance and superiority, which quickly meets with rejection from other group participants and thus reinforces the prejudices of the narcissistically structured patients. Here, a great deal of sensitivity and moderation on the part of the group leadership is needed.

Example

Over the years, I have treated some young men individually who suffered from significant narcissistic deficits. Their lack of self-esteem, which was synonymous with a difficult positioning in reality and with attachment problems, also in relation to work activities, was usually tried to be compensated by carefully hidden fantasies of their own greatness and significance. On the basis of this dynamic, a tremendous anger and much hatred lurked, which reflected in the countertransference, i.e., the perception of the patients by the therapists, in the form of boredom, fatigue, and dissatisfaction. At some point, I decided with several of these patients to apply for an analytical group following the individual analysis, as a combination treatment with occasional individual sessions between the groups. The narcissistic defense of these patients became apparent in the group in a way that had not been noticeable before. They appeared arrogant, largely ignored the contact offers of the other group participants. Similarly structured co-patients were antagonized. However, due to the fanning out of the transference and the previous and parallel individual treatment, the patients had usually developed so much frustration tolerance and a lesser vulnerability that they learned to deal with the sometimes annoying group members. Their anger calmed down, they came to the groups quite gladly over time, then increasingly spoke empathetically about themselves and with the others. ◄

These changes could be explained by assuming that so many positive introjects could be built up that the affect- and self-regulation could be improved to such an extent that at least the greatest affect storms of the "narcissistic rage" could be better endured. In this way, they were confronted with their own aggressiveness in a way that before was often unfamiliar to them. Slowly, many succeeded in better aligning their perception of others with their self-perception. If this does not succeed, it can happen that patients abruptly leave the group, or there are heated verbal disputes. To understand how this can happen and also to avoid it as much as possible, we need to deal more deeply with the phenomenon of narcissism, as it underlies many of today's psychodynamics (see Chap. 11)

References

Dalal, F (1998) Taking the group seriously. Jessica Kingsley Publishers, London

Frischenschlager, O (2011) Arndt, P, Klingen, N: Psychosomatik und Psychotherapie. Psychotherapie-Wissenschaft, 1(2), 145. https://psychotherapie-wissenschaft.info/article/view/235 (Stand: 16.9.2023)

Giegerich, W (2012) What is Soul? Spring Journal Books, New Orleans

Illouz, E (2016) Warum Liebe weh tut. Suhrkamp, Berlin

Jung, C G (1995) Gesammelte Werke, 9/1. Walter, Düsseldorf

Kohut, H (1989) Wie heilt die Psychoanalyse. Suhrkamp, Frankfurt

Lesmeister, R (2017) Begehren, Schuld und Neubeginn. Psychosozial Verlag, Gießen

Money-Kyrle, R (1971) The aim of psychoanalysis. International Journal of Psychoanalysis 52: 103–106

Stern, D (2018) Der Gegenwartsmoment. Brandes & Apsel Verlag, Frankfurt/M

Türk, D (2020) Einzel- und Gruppenpsychotherapie als Kombinations- und Verbundtherapie – ein Erfahrungsbericht aus der Praxis. Gruppenpsychother. Gruppendynamik 56: 151–171

Yalom, I (2005) Die Schopenhauer-Kur. btb-verlag, München

Special Patient Groups

11

Abstract

This chapter discusses the prerequisites and special treatment interventions for more severe forms of mental disorders in groups. This includes patients with narcissistic structures, traumatized patients, and patients at risk of addiction. The assumed setting is that these patients are treated in mixed, analytical groups with other types of disorders. Special difficulties and variations will be examined. It turns out that under certain conditions, even more severe personality accentuations or disorders can indeed achieve an improvement in symptoms and a gain in structure within this framework.

11.1 Narcissistic Patients in Groups

When treating narcissistic patients in groups, it makes a difference whether you are dealing with younger or older patients. In middle age, the psychological structures are often so entrenched that the surrender of grandiose fantasies, the confrontation with finiteness and limitations, as is the case for these people, is capable of triggering such shame and rage that participation in a group can be quite strenuous for both the affected individuals and the other group members. After all, it is about these people giving up the worldview they have maintained, almost admitting to themselves that they have been on the wrong track so far. The unconscious view of the narcissistic person, being someone very special, does not come from a particular malice or arrogance, even if it can often seem that way. Rather, they cannot accept that others might like them as they are, accept them, want to share commonalities with them.

V. Münch, *Group Experience as a Resource*,
https://doi.org/10.1007/978-3-662-70864-4_11

Example

A now middle-aged patient had already shown a dismissive, degrading attitude towards peers of the same sex since childhood and adolescence. He learned to live withdrawn in his worlds of thought and had little real contact, was hardly in groups or clubs, did not play team sports. This attitude was an internalized identification with the aggressor, as he himself was seen very one-sidedly and with little empathy by his parents. He always had the feeling that he should conform to the roles or images of his parents, less so that his own needs, emotions, and ideas were assigned any value. This development eventually led him into a social profession. With this, he associated the idea that he could identify there not "classically male", but rather with "soft" ideals, such as empathy, sensitivity, permeability, and imaginative activity, which he perceived as more femininely connoted. This was another attempt to escape the attributions from the outside, but as expected, it also led to problems. Only very gradually was the patient able to penetrate this psychodynamic and better accept his inner misery and distress, which helped, to significantly relativize his narcissistic grandiose ideas. ◀

It is often a very slow and laborious process for these patients when they gradually realize that they can reduce their efforts to be admired and just be there. It is also the greatest success in the treatment of narcissistic people when they learn to accept themselves with their personal gifts and weaknesses as average, normal people and do not have to torment the others in a group with their anyway unfulfillable needs. It is always the same: everything is already there. It becomes increasingly clear that there is nothing to do, one is part of a group, one belongs, one does not need to make oneself smaller or larger than one is. This can be a profound, transformative experience for someone who has had little positive experience in and with groups in childhood. Suddenly it becomes clear what has always been missing. And it is bitter to acknowledge that one has done a lot for a long time to avoid perhaps getting it retrospectively. The narcissistic rage, which arises from the humiliation of unfulfilled desires, is usually good at driving others away and making oneself permanently unpopular. Thus, the narcissistic person is in a spiral from which they can hardly find a way out. I have already described my experiences with narcissistic patients in groups in more detail elsewhere, I just want to note the most important points here (see Münch 2016).

The Dynamics of Narcissistic Disorder

Narcissism is a good measure for describing our varying relationships to groups. Pathological narcissism and healthy group experience are almost mutually exclusive. Why is that? Neville Symington (1999), an Australian colleague, has associated narcissistic developments with these people's refusal of the "life-giver". He understood this to be an unconscious refusal to be able to make oneself dependent on others. The loss of autonomy and self-determination is feared. But so one loses the connection to vital inner drives and emotions, i.e., one's own liveliness in large areas. Life becomes something willed, made, which can make everyday life very strenuous. These people lack the experience that they are seen, perceived, and appreciated in the presence and exchange with others and do not lose anything, but rather can gain something if they move in groups. Thus, they never find rest and relief from their inner struggles, which all revolve around the issues of recognition, self-esteem, and existential fear. Even more difficult for them is to learn to accept that they are always and everywhere involved in groups and dependent on other people.

The Narcissism of Society

Thus, a circle closes: The postmodern society promotes narcissism in the sense of self-realization and a "me-first-thinking" (cf. Illouz 2016; Maaz 2014; Hardt 2019). At the same time, it provides means such as therapies to counteract and mitigate this tendency. In the (individual) treatments, the paradox emerges that patients often complain about not being able to assert themselves enough, articulate themselves, or even perceive themselves. This must be taken very seriously at first, as patients usually suffer from the fact that they were indeed mirrored and empathetically accompanied too little by their early caregivers. This usually leads to a reversal of concern: The children become "parentified" while they are actually in great emotional distress. This has a permanently damaging effect on the personality structure. In individual therapy, these people understandably often appear very needy (depressive processing) or demanding (narcissistic processing). They want their counterpart, the treating person, all to themselves. Therefore, they are usually very resistant to group therapy at the beginning. They have the idea that they should again, as with their parents, listen to and endure the stories of troubled people without having the opportunity to react and take a position. Both are frightening: the fear that the personal story repeats itself and no change takes place, but also the opportunity to position oneself, to show oneself is frightening. Because these people have no experience with this. They must fear that others cannot accept and endure their feelings, including aggressive feelings.

Alternative Experiences

This is exactly where the opportunity arises to make an alternative experience in reality by participating in a group. Slowly and in small steps, it can be shown that one's own fears do not have to come true and that a completely different, more conflict-capable, but therefore also more trusting relationship can be built with the fellow participants. How can this trust be established, even though the narcissistic patients make it quite difficult to like them and enjoy working with them? At least three factors are, in my opinion, decisive:

a) Negative Capability—the term, which goes back to the English poet John Keats (1817), describes the ability to endure uncertainty and not knowing. The term was adopted by Bion and introduced into psychoanalysis.
b) Patience—as a psychoanalyst who sometimes conducts treatments over a very long period, usually at least 3–4 years, the observation that changes often take

a long time is a daily experience. This is especially true in connection with narcissistic disorders of patients and in group processes: If the unconscious of the patients has enough time to unfold and is not forced into retreat by the fear of an imminent end of treatment, then long-suppressed, unconscious contents and conflicts unfold, which then become visible in the therapeutic relationships. Abuse experiences are also often remembered only years after the start of therapy.

c) Humor—especially in connection with the treatment of narcissism, humor is a decisive therapeutic variable. The high vulnerability of narcissistic people also makes them very humorless people. Which in turn is detrimental to the ability to cope adequately with reality and also to the effect on other people. So if such a patient laughs (about himself) and integrates humor into his affect repertoire, then a lot is gained. The lack of humor and the false seriousness of the imagined own superiority are the exact opposite of this.

Example

Especially in traumatized patients, a so-called psychological skin is often missing, which makes them very vulnerable to injuries in a regressed state. Thus, a group can also potentially have a retraumatizing character. I have sometimes experienced with patients that they reported very angrily and disturbed about groups in an inpatient context, which were perhaps led by not yet sufficiently experienced colleagues. One patient told me that she had been virtually forced to make statements, even though she felt very uncomfortable. Unfortunately, it is not a rare exception that groups in clinics are led by people who have neither sufficient self-experience nor group leadership experience, but this should change soon with the reform of psychotherapist training in Germany, which obligatorily includes group training. ◄

11.2 Trauma and Group

In groups, patients are reminded of their vulnerability and also finiteness through the stories of others, but also through inquiries about their own unmentioned experiences, aspects that are often barely bearable for traumatized and narcissistic patients. At the beginning of every group there is fear, even among conductors. A group first needs a psychological skin, it must “close” before it can be perceived as protective. This in turn reminds us of the analogy of the imagination of the group as a maternal, protective space.

Traumas in Analytical Individual and Group Therapy

The effects of the protective and inspiring character of groups become concrete in the increasing interaction of the participants, their also increasing openness, which is further promoted in the suggestions for self-reflection and more precise perception of communication and interaction in the group. Through the realization of sharing common problem themes and also the emerging will and optimism to be able to solve them better together, the group process gradually gets underway. In this process, initial, "naive" ideas about the way in which a group is helpfully effective are gradually transformed. One distances oneself from the expectation of receiving concrete instructions for action and "tips", and enters into a process of mutual storytelling, questioning, and begins to suspect that the answers to the inner questions could come about in a completely different form than originally thought. Trauma patients need a particularly protected space. In this respect, they also need a certain stability and resilience before they can be admitted to an analytical group. The situation is different in the topic-related closed groups often offered in clinics, which often run very structured, sometimes also have a psychoeducational character. Supportive individual sessions are usually necessary in any case. Franziska Hennigsen (2012) has convincingly shown that analytical individual psychotherapy can be very effective in the treatment of severe traumas. It would be desirable if there could be a corresponding study for analytical group psychotherapy.

11.3 Addicted Patients in Groups

When approaching outpatient psychotherapeutic treatment of people at risk of addiction or those already addicted, there are several points to consider. Apart from the fact that in this case in Germany a period of abstinence of at least one year must be observed before psychotherapy can be applied for, the popular format of group therapy in addiction work itself poses some obstacles that are often overlooked. In Germany, a distinction is made between addiction therapy and psychotherapy. Severely addicted people are required to first complete a longer withdrawal treatment in a specialized facility. This can also be done on an outpatient basis, but not in a practice. Afterwards, these patients, as well as those with moderate to lighter problems, i.e., at the level of substance abuse, can turn to an outpatient psychotherapy practice. If there is an abstinent or proven controlled handling of the addictive substance, group psychotherapy can theoretically also be a method of choice. The stability sought by addicted people in the form of rituals, a familiar environment, and a safe and comforting environment can be positively answered by groups with the quality they provide.

The Group as a Symbol for the Stable, Nurturing Mother

The background for the dynamics of addicted people, but generally all orally needy patients, is the following situation in the primary family: People who are often structurally deficient often have little to no continuous bonding experience. They are often materially spoiled, but emotionally very neglected. The great attraction of addictive substances comes, among other things, from the immense unconscious longings for early oral care and sometimes also prenatal, paradisiacally associated states. However, people who are disappointed in their early dyadic relationship experience and unconsciously often very angry are quickly overwhelmed by groups. The often changing participants and sometimes also changing therapists in addiction work constellate those unstable, little secure bonding constellations that must be considered as the starting point of the patients' problems. However, group capability or a sufficient ability to triangulate cannot yet function in people who can often hardly achieve and maintain a sufficient internal subject-object separation. This means that many addicted people perceive their environment and their fellow human beings as not sufficiently separated from themselves. Their lack of experience with concrete interaction partners, with an "opposite", causes enormous mistrust of new reference persons, so that initially the dyadic experience is at the forefront of treatment. As a rule, a longer individual contact is therefore necessary to establish sufficient stability of the relationship.

The Group in Competition with the Addictive Substance

In addition, in these treatments, it is necessary to ensure regular verification of abstinence by means of blood values. However, this represents a special case in the psychotherapeutic field. Most analytical colleagues have little motivation to treat this group of patients due to bad experiences with the ability to abstain and also the lack of cooperation in the groups and the ever-present risk of relapse. However, I was able to get to know some patients with a secondary, less pronounced tendency towards substance abuse. They benefited from the groups, but were usually unable to work on their issues, as they were foreign to the other group participants. All my early attempts, however, to treat more severely addicted patients in a group, after an appropriate period of abstinence and with credible motivation, ultimately failed with relapses and dropouts. Here, one should take the indication seriously and refrain from premature treatment, even if patients can win you over in a very urgent and skilled manner. Perhaps the desired triangulation, the confrontation with more than two different actors in the group, often fails so badly because the addictive substance is experienced as part of the personality. But this already occupies two positions of the three psychic actors: with the patient and the addictive substance. Especially a group then quickly overwhelms the concerned.

References

Hennigsen, F (2012) Psychoanalysen mit traumatisierten Patienten. Klett-Cotta, Stuttgart

Hardt, J (2019) Psychoanalyse im Widerstreit mit der digitalen Welt. Psyche 73,9: 826–851

Illouz, E (2016) Warum Liebe weh tut. Suhrkamp, Berlin

Maaz, H J (2014) Die narzisstische Gesellschaft. dtv, München

Münch, V (2016) Der narzisstische Patient in der Gruppe. In: Schimkus, M, Stuck, U (2016) Selbst, Ich und Wir. Brandes & Apsel Verlag, Frankfurt/M

Symington, N (1999) Narzissmus. Psychosozial-Verlag, Gießen

12 Group Developments

Abstract

A group process is not a linear process. And the development of the group is different from the development of the individual group participants within it. Both dimensions intertwine, especially when it comes to a semi-open group. The individual phases of group development, from initial fears and projections to more trust and confidence, but also to increased conflict resolution skills, are relatively well described (see Yalom, Theory and Practice of Group Psychotherapy. Klett-Cotta, Stuttgart, 2016). However, there are also destructive developments in groups that deserve attention (see Nitsun, The Anti-Group. Routledge, London, 2014). No group is self-sustaining and will only bring about beneficial and creative aspects. It always involves the acceptance of the shadow, the acceptance of loneliness, of emptiness, of anger and destructive desire. We will get to know the concept of the "Anti-Group" and how well it is suited to describe the polarity of development in and of groups. Various fears, which can revolve around injuries, shame, and sexuality, must first be recognized before they can block the group process less strongly. Communication is something that every group must develop and build anew, always with the help of the personal resources and also limits of its members. Beyond all resistances, there are also archetypal forces that have a positive influence on the group process. These forces and the question of how they can be used by the leadership of a group will be examined in more depth in Chap. 14 and 15.

12.1 The Course of Groups

Example

Recently, I initiated a new group. In the first session, everyone, including the therapist, was nervous. The uncertainty was evident in various scenarios,

V. Münch, *Group Experience as a Resource*,
https://doi.org/10.1007/978-3-662-70864-4_12

themes, and situations: For one, several participants tested the framework by arriving late to the group session for different reasons. The two participants whom I considered the most anxious and severely ill sat next to me, as if they were seeking security. In different ways, the image of a mother who has to be there for her children was invoked thematically. Transferred to the group, the question arose whether one could get enough here. The question of trust also arose. It was described with the still paranoid fantasy that one could not be sure whether someone was eavesdropping on the group with their mobile phone. This led to a recap of the group rules regarding this issue (phones off!), but also reflected the theme. Another aspect of this initial group session was the fear of becoming dependent on the help of others or the therapist. This was evident in that someone had to keep their mobile phone in their hand throughout the session. Confronted with this, he brought a stone to the next session to keep his hands busy and reduce his immense tensions. Soon he began to tell… The group tried to conjure itself: We can do this, it's hard, but it will probably be worth it. Finally, it became clear who needed the most support in the group at this time, a patient told a short personal vignette. ◂

12.2 The Anti-Group

A concept used to better understand destructive processes in groups is that of the "Anti-Group" by the recently deceased British psychoanalyst Morris Nitsun (2014). He is concerned with the acceptance of these impulses and forces and the constant work on aggression, which can often also subtly negatively affect the development of groups. Ultimately, as a conductor, one needs a relationship with these destructive forces in order to enable a process of transformation for the group and the individual group participants. All too often, group processes are depicted as too one-sidedly favorable, development-promoting, and overall rather idealistic. But it is precisely this one-sided idealization that can lead to the disintegration of groups. C. G. Jung described this dynamic as the principle of opposition: If an existing force is suppressed in favor of another, this unconsciously and in the end strengthens the influence of the unwanted forces. So if a group wants to please the leader too much and "reward" with "progress" and new insights, this comes at the expense of integrating the resentments and transferences existing against him or her. If the participants do not get to know the shadow aspects of their psychological life sufficiently, they are not sensitized to their unconsciously controlling influence and must submit to the compulsion to repeat.

The Interaction of Constructive and Destructive Forces

Nitsun is interested in how positive, constructive, and connecting forces on the one hand, and destructive, divisive, thus negatively connoted forces on the other hand, coexist and interact in groups to achieve an appropriate, realistic therapeutic goal. He assumes that one is always in the field of tension between these poles of force. He also concedes to the feelings connoted as negative that they contribute to keeping a group together. If these are sufficiently well held, endured, and communicated, this is an opportunity for the participants to take away a more complete picture of their own inner world. Smith and Berg (1988) also assume that there can be no groups without conflicts and that progression and regression alternate, there is always isolation *and* connection, bonding *and* alienation. On the one hand, a group makes individual fates in groups visible up to this point, on the other hand, it always offers the chance for a new design of this fate, as a broader, deeper view of it is established when the different perspectives come together. But still, the problem arises that group phenomena appear less tangible, more unpredictable, more ambiguous than we often like. This not only scares patients, but also many of us, as the relatively small proportion of group analysts shows.

Example

In the initial phase of one of my early groups, well over half of the participants were significantly depressed, which in my view was due to the fact that many had been severely traumatized in their childhood. I had paid less attention to whether there might have been positive group experiences here and there before I started the group. In the first half year, it proved to be extremely difficult at times to motivate the group to work constructively. I was often met with an impenetrable silence, triggered by fears and mistrust. No one was willing to take the first step and reveal something about themselves and their life situation. I countered this resistance with a kind of psychoeducation and group interpretations, which were intended to improve understanding of the current group situation. Finally, a discussion ignited on the topic of "cancellation fees". Anger and unwillingness were expressed. After that, something seemed to have loosened up and more was told. A great deal of empathy and patience was needed before this group "learned to walk", i.e., the participants were willing to initiate contact with others on their own. Here I needed a lot of what is often described as the integrating function of the leader: I tried to explain, to mediate, to show resonance in a difficult situation that probably corresponded to the atmosphere of many of the parents' homes, as it had been perceived by several participants. Unconsciously, these people recreated their childhood situation in the group anew. The aggression also had to first constellate and show itself. The defense stemmed from the initial identification with the aggressor and initially prevented new, more constructive and healing experiences from being made. ◄

There are many signs of the presence of the so-called anti-group tendency: Verbal attacks on the leader or other group participants, frequent absences, sometimes also somatic illnesses and therapy dropouts are signs that individual participants become carriers of this anti-mood rampant in every group. In such situations, it is important to understand the individual as a carrier of desires and fears that are updated in the group and not to allow scapegoat dynamics. Healthy groups that rather integrate the anti-group impulse react integratively to acting out: they show surprise, disappointment and anger when someone unexpectedly wants to leave the group, but often quickly return to business as usual. This may be healthy, but it also avoids the experience of loss and abandonment. If a member does not fit into the group at all, a dropout can also strengthen cohesion. Groups often understand very well whether it is a loss or a gain when someone drops out. In general, disappointment and frustration in the group are better absorbed when the inevitability of such events and thus contradictions and limitations are emphasized. According to Bion (1991), the anti-group would be a failure of the "container-contained" at the group level. Due to excessive fear in the group, it regresses to developmentally earlier defense mechanisms. Individual, non-integrated aggression is thus more easily channeled and the anti-group gives it expression by directing this individual aggression towards the group itself. Such regressed groups no longer possess any creative, constructive potential. Since Bion's view of the group is quite negative here, the question arises as to what constructive group characteristics there are. Because a beneficial group dynamic is much more than the absence of archaic defense processes. If we look more closely, the process in the group does not only take place between the poles of constructiveness and destructiveness, but also between the polarity of presence and absence, which is always given in therapies and relationships. If group participants come into contact with the feeling of missing the group, for example during vacations, of feeling abandoned and alone, then a bond is forming.

Winnicott's Incommunicado: Areas of the Uncommunicable

The resistance to opening up can have reasons other than the dynamics of the anti-group. Winnicott's (1988) concept of "Incommunicado" points out that there is an area in every person that someone is neither willing nor able to provide information about. This innermost area of the self must sometimes remain unconscious even for the individuals concerned. It is important that this should not be seen as a resistance to be overcome, and therefore any pressure on patients towards self-disclosure would be inappropriate. It is not about the area of the unconscious, which is considered the dynamic unconscious. It is about, with Lesmeister (2009), never losing sight of respect for the patient's resistance. The intensity and rigidity of the aggressive expression of individuals must be regulated and commented on within groups. As a rule, this then also leads to an increased feeling that the group can become a place for growth and security. My experience is that a certain relief sets in when someone in a group critically comments on the behavior of another on their behalf. Most often, patients become the target of such criticism when they either a) rarely or never participate, b) often complain and tell long-winded stories, but then hardly respond to the objections of others, or c) mainly express themselves with "advice" on the problems of others. All these reactions have in common that the individuals concerned thereby withdraw from direct emotional involvement and relation to the other person. It can trigger intense aggression when corresponding complexes in the "instructed" are triggered. However, in the holding, supporting environment of a functioning group, the clarification of this dynamic is helpful and takes everyone a step further. Those who are reacted to aversively, in the best case, recognize the aggression as something of their own, defended, the group experiences itself as courageous in confrontation, trusting in the supporting matrix of relationships in the group.

The Defense of the Group Leadership

Group conductors also have anti-group components. But they should know these. Otherwise, it could be that individual group participants act out exactly these destructive tendencies. After I had to experience how colleagues who had previously led groups eventually gave up this activity, I began to think about the causes. In the descriptions, working in the group was extremely tedious due to the destruction of the participants. Over time, I got the impression that they themselves had no motivation to offer groups anymore, as they seemed to be constantly working against the resistance of the patients. On the side of the therapists, an almost compulsive identification with the positive, constructive pole was noticeable. They described themselves as if they were constantly devalued and "devoured" by the group, without getting anything in return. Perhaps an misunderstood anti-group dynamic was at work here.

However, when groups often complain about others, society, I soon ask what exactly makes the group so angry. Usually, many closer triggers are then found, which turn out to be more understandable and influenceable. If there are frequent dropouts, as was the case at the beginning of my group work, I initially missed interpreting these aggressive acts as an expression of the dynamics of the group and thus also of the others. I was relieved to find that the groups continued to work. Group interpretations can be relieving in the context of processing aggressive feelings. The group as such can thus lead individuals out of personal feelings of guilt when aggressive tendencies are recognized as widespread and not reprehensible. At the same time, group interpretations also lead in a further step to the trail of the various personal sources of dissatisfaction and resentment.

12.3 Failed Communication

In trauma patients, there can be a lot of fear of voicing distressing experiences, as there is often little real positive experience with others and many unconscious fantasies have been developed. To be forced to arrange with physical closeness, the presence of others, from which one may not be able to retreat to the extent one is used to in everyday life, —this too can cause a lot of stress in group therapy. Verbal communication also causes fear, there is the fear of the spoken word, which seems to have a kind of finality. In addition, some words must remain limited: There are unspeakable things beyond functioning defense: Things that one must consider at work, but must accept in silence. There is unspeakable, unthinkable for everyone at any time. Considering this is important for the group conductors. But also the group participants often gain surprisingly quickly an intuitive security in the delicate handling with traumatized and very sensitive fellow patients. Some participants are tragically entangled in their inability to communicate appropriately. They project mental contents, create rejection and confusion in others and thus cannot experience real encounter and relief through contact. Then one sometimes has to interrupt the situation. Some patients, who can still endure the individual session, come under a lot of pressure in the group. For them it is wrong if they feel they have to talk in any case. Initially, it is usually about preverbal, simple existence. Ultimately, according to Nitsun (2014), groups are primarily about attunement—an important term from research on early communication between mother and child. It describes the importance of the ability of caregivers to tune into a child and its emotions, to resonate. Without sufficient care in this relationship, a small person remains internally orphaned and yet has to somehow cope with his inner, emotional world. In groups, according to Nitsun, a lot happens already at this level. But if there are too few participants in a group who can empathize appropriately because they are also deprived, this can also have a retraumatizing effect. Then it can happen that someone complains about always being criticized, and thus makes the group helpless and incapacitates it. This too is ultimately an anti-group effect.

On a deeper level, the group process always initially involves the translation of non-metabolized, psychic contents into more conscious, verbalized units, but sometimes also primarily about containment. Thematically, it is initially about dependency needs and fears of appropriation, then about autonomy and assertion of one's own interests, finally about enduring a multi-person perspective, the ability to triangulate, which can be seen in connection with the oedipal basic conflict and whose non-achievement is strongly associated with blocked inner creativity and productivity.

Example

A group participant told me in a one-on-one conversation about a sexual assault in her youth. However, she never found the courage to report this experience in the group. Nevertheless, she showed herself increasingly self-confident and resilient in her external contacts and also in the group context. The reactions of the other group participants to her led me to suspect that they had unconscious knowledge of what was discussed in the relevant individual session. This development shows that it is by no means always necessary for everything to be spoken out in order to develop changing power. Through the changed view of the treating person, a space may also have opened up from which the patient benefited. Perhaps it was significant for her to be allowed to once set boundaries with the transferred father figure against the group perceived as a demanding mother with a secret. Her biography certainly suggested this thought. ◄

12.4 Fears and Their Defense in Groups

In therapeutic groups, there is often a high idealization of the leaders or conductors (see Chapt. 13) in the initial phase. The participants regress to early wishful thinking, making the reactions more emotional and also more childlike. Bion

(1991) argued that it is primarily the participants' fears of their own fragmentation and annihilation that are triggered in unstructured groups and also psychologically combated with typical defense mechanisms. These elemental fears unconsciously trigger sometimes violent aggressions, which in turn are projected onto the group as such, as they are experienced by the individuals as difficult to bear. The group becomes a threatening and persecuting object. In this post-Kleinian view, represented by both Bion and subsequently Nitsun, the occurrence of anti-group phenomena is also a result of aggressive partial objects projected into the group, i.e., unbearable, own inner parts of the participants. "Evil" is no longer projected outward (the group complains about other groups), but is suspected within the group itself. Likewise, repressed images of the primal scene (the parents having sex) can be perceived as aggression, thus shaping fantasies and burdening the group process.

Everyone Can Also Experience Themselves as Helpful and Competent
It is known that these intense reactions are partly favored by a group framework that assigns a very exposed and abstinent role to the leader. In my experience, groups differ greatly depending on how active and authentic the conductors are present in it. In my opinion, a combination of regressive, reactualizing, and progressive, constructive impulses is helpful for promoting a vitalizing group process as such. This is exactly where the basic character of a group comes in handy: Since the participants all bring different experiences and can be seen as wounded or already further developed at different points of their psyche, the chance of help and support from others is greater even in difficult moments. The respective different needs always point complementarily to different resources for coping with psychological tensions. In other words: Everyone can contribute their own positive experiences as an "expert" in a different area. This process is typical for a functioning group. At the beginning of a group that is still unfamiliar, complaints are sometimes simply followed by the complaints of others. Unconsciously, the therapists are thus addressed as fantasized omnipotent helper figures. It is about the anger of the abandoned and undersupplied. The past is psychologically revived.

Unconscious Envy
In Kleinian psychoanalysis, the unconscious envy effect is attributed a major role in the development of psychological tensions. This can also lead to the described anti-group phenomena. Envy can be directed at intellectual or external features, often it is also an expression of different social origin (cf. Dalal 1998). Participants who develop more slowly can envy others for their progress. Ultimately, it is about thematizing and accepting this envy. After all, envy can also contain a hint of hitherto untrodden developmental paths (cf. Kast 1996). Often then shame effects come up. Envy avoidance can also be caused by a negative therapeutic reaction. Thus, development is prevented, as otherwise envy could arise in others, be it in the group or outside. In addition, the often envied therapist is tried to be punished unconsciously.

Example

In a stationary addiction therapy facility, a colleague experienced how a destructive dynamic unfolded and brought down the entire facility. The different payment of psychologists, doctors on the one hand, and so-called ex-users, i.e., trained former drug addicts, on the other hand, generated intense envy and hatred. The psychologists were subtly disadvantaged, cut off from information, not integrated into the team. When a conflict between patients and therapists escalated, it turned out that many of the non-academically trained forces of the facility had narcissistically, sexually, and monetarily abused patients for years. There were sexual relationships between therapists and patients, mutual dependencies that made any treatment a farce! If there was a risk that these power relations could be exposed, the weaker patients were "thrown" out of the facility on a large scale, often simply left to their fate on the street. The facility was soon closed, as this completely ruined its reputation. ◄

12.5 Interpersonal Complications and Fear of Shame

As already mentioned, many people prefer individual treatment over group treatment. They protect themselves from revealing their desires for closeness and connection in the group and from being disappointed. This also attempts to obtain a kind of reparation for a disappointing one-on-one relationship in childhood. The idea of complicated relationships, of confusion and (sibling) competition, and the necessity to have to share in the group (to have participation as a "participant") can further intensify these primary desires. Often, the desires for exclusivity of the relationship are directed towards the conductor, they are intensified by transferences. If these desires are ultimately disappointed, this can intensify anti-group reactions. The group is identified with the leaving, disappointing primary object. Prognostically favorable are at least a basis of good primary relationship experiences, preferably even in groups (kindergarten, friends, school). Then it is significant that positive experiences can be collected in the therapeutic group soon after its start. Whether it is that the containing and the moderation of the fantasies and affects are provided by the person in charge, or that coalitions also form among the participants to reduce fear. If a group member can hardly interact with the others due to his social special position, a scapegoat position can also develop from this. Therefore, it is usually attempted to always include at least two people with closer thematic or biographical similarities (Noah's Ark principle). Occasionally, this also corresponds to a psychopathological or typological (cf. Chap. 15) classification.

12.6 Sexuality

According to Nitsun, the unconscious defense of affects associated with the primal scene fantasy can also trigger an anti-group dynamic. Thus, the fantasies about the unity of the family, the ideas of sexuality and corresponding sexual fears, as well as fantasies about their creative or destructive qualities would be aroused. The author mainly refers to individual psychological and also classical psychoanalytic ideas and does not take into account the many other relevant group formations. At least it follows that the conductors should also have a corresponding openness to these topics, so that arrested fantasies and ideas can be set in motion. The topic of sexuality is the most difficult in groups, as many archaic ideas about aggression are associated with it. Sexuality has something irritating, boundary-breaking, frightening, which many people then process regressively. If a group is very fixated on the "anti-libidinal ego" because it is afraid of strong affects, then it is also robbed of the energy necessary for growth.

Example

Male patients who had to experience the father's violence against the mother as a child often find it very difficult to identify with the male, paternal, for fear that they could then no longer control their perpetrator parts. If the father has been verbally or physically intrusive, one does not want to be "like that" at all, but often also avoids one's own assertive, self-assertive life expressions, which can lead to "dwindling" biographies. Behind this is a too shame-laden, inhibited personality development. Sometimes this dynamic leads to the general avoidance of contacts and especially partnership relationships. In groups, successive suggestions and examples from others can contribute to gradually dissolving this defense. ◂

12.7 Ideals and Their Unattainability

A main characteristic of narcissism (see Sect. 11.1) is the excessively high self-ideal of those affected. The conditions of today's society also contribute to this. In a podcast of the SRF series "Sternstunden der Philosophie", the philosopher Isolde Charim (2023) speaks of the self-ideal as the "representative of society in our psyche", which puts the psyche under unprecedented pressure, as it is no longer about defending oneself against external pressure and threat, but against a part of one's own person. It can be stated in advance that the necessary work of de-idealization of the treatment takes place almost incidentally in a psychotherapy group. This even applies to the conductors, insofar as they must always make illusory ideas about the patients due to never complete knowledge of them, before the process teaches them better. This also particularly affects the individual path that patients choose when it comes to how they deal with their problems and burdens as well as conflicts after they have addressed these in the treatments. Often enough, the developments initiated in therapies also surprise the therapists themselves. And this is a good thing. Because then they can honestly rejoice in increased decision-making ability and increased joy of life and do not have to hide their disappointment that the patients do not take the path they suspected.

The necessary failure at the ideals, Charim continues in the above-mentioned podcast, leads to the ego being repeatedly referred to its inadequacy. However, the defining feeling of the time is that one must "become more". Peter Sloterdijk (2009) has also dealt extensively with this topic in his book *You Must Change Your Life*. Our patients also move in this field of conflict, beyond all individual shaping of this topic.

The Group Experiences Itself as Creative

In addition to competition and rivalry, groups create the new experience for many that constructive and trust-building elements are being built through the joint witnessing of the emotional reality of others. To put it bluntly: The more intense the processing of negatively connoted emotions, the more trust can be built. The mutual exploration of sensitivity leads to increased resilience (see Flaßpöhler 2021). This can also lead to the self-esteem, the feeling of self-worth, arising again or sometimes for the first time. This is then not identified with the promises of salvation of a world of social media dependent on quantification and rankings. The comparison among each other in the therapy group inevitably includes the otherwise hidden levels of the repressed and unconscious. This is perceived by the group and usually reflected back in a tolerable form, so that a different, more comprehensive perspective gradually emerges for the individuals,—on others, the world and especially on themselves.

Example

The fact that the effect of a group can sometimes take place very quietly and yet point to deeper processes of de-idealization can be discovered in different ways time and again: A patient who had long expressed skepticism about participating in a group and who showed extreme shyness in the group, began to take an interest in others. This was initially only visible in her gaze and with an occasional smile. At some point, her statements also clearly showed that she was indeed dealing with the stories of the other group participants, contrary to the external impression. The hitherto overwhelming conviction that the lives of others had little to offer her was cautiously re-examined. It became clear that the patient had put on a defensive, cool-looking "shell" out of great inner fear. The background was traumatic experiences, violence, flight, and narcissistic abuse. ◄

12.8 Meeting of the Group Outside the Therapeutic Framework

When I participated in my first analytical group in the 1980s, we made it a habit to go to the nearby Greek restaurant after therapy. Although the analyst did not like this, it was not explicitly forbidden. Maybe we would have done it anyway? The subsequent entanglements among the participants at that time suggest from today's perspective that a stricter framework would have been necessary.

In my own groups, I handle the topic in such a way that I address it and try to justify why it is important to bring everything that happens between the participants outside the therapy session back into the group to make it discussable there. When I then see how the group participants stand together in the square in front of the practice while I go home, I have to endure my jealousy on the one hand, and tolerate what they are doing there on the other. Meanwhile, I am pleased that the group members seem to feel comfortable with each other, some of what connects them, I think, is thanks to these moments of encounter between "door and hinge", before or after the group session. In the group sessions themselves, on the other hand, the power of transference and the pressing and contradictory feelings are palpable. This contrast can also be interpreted accordingly.

Reflection instead of control
Ultimately, as a therapist, I have to admit: I am unable to control everything and I don't even have to, because usually it is constructive, creative impulses that are exchanged, gestures of humanity, of closeness. These then recede into the background again in the sessions under the influence of dynamics, transference, and resistance. But my impression is that it can make the group easier if you can get the impression that the others are all just normal people and not just people with serious problems. I think of several decades-long friendships that grew out of my own group self-experiences. Today I can see that even the "strict" therapist could not have everything on her radar. This had both advantages and disadvantages.

No fear of groups
The urge to exchange without the therapists is not surprising, because in hardly any other context do people show themselves so openly and vulnerably and have similar goals for themselves: suffer less, have fewer symptoms, understand themselves, learn to accept themselves. My group participants often do not know any other people than the "problem-laden" ones from their group (besides the problem-laden ones from their environment) for a long time before they slowly start to look around more in the world. It can also happen that group participants join together and criticize their group therapists. If individuals feel too vulnerable, they try to form coalitions in this way. Usually, these developments can be interpreted and resolved well when the fear has decreased. I am aware that it always remains an illusion, beyond any fantasy of completeness, to be able to "know everything" about patients. They always have to hide deeply unconscious thoughts of

themselves from themselves, also from me, regardless of all possibilities of empathy. Knausgard (2020) described this in the novel *Out of the World* with the words: "But the thought is beautiful: that there are things about us that we consider unique and therefore tell no human soul. Things that we all know and to which we all remain silent." (ibid., p. 59). How and why patients react so differently in groups and why it is important to gather many different people with different topics in a group, yes also different generations, I will try to outline more precisely in Chap. 14 and 15.

All these thoughts about the group processes can give one the necessary serenity that is important for group work. With Mattke and Strauß (2009), it is about "no longer having to fear groups" for participants, but also for the conductors alike on different levels.

References

Bion, W R (1991) Erfahrungen in Gruppen. Fischer, Frankfurt/M
Charim, I (2023) Wie narzisstisch ist unsere Gesellschaft? Podcast Sternstunden der Philosophie vom 14.1.2023, https://open.spotify.com/episode/3RdAZOJYIqOA0DVy7UZIJR?si=B9BF8C9B-B08B-4433-908D-F71B2FF58399&utm_source=system-ua-share&nd=1 (Stand: 17.09.2023)
Dalal, F (1998) Taking the group seriously. Jessica Kingsley Publishers
Flaßpöhler, S (2021) Sensibel. Klett-Cotta, Stuttgart
Kast, V (1996) Neid und Eifersucht. Walter, Düsseldorf
Knausgard, K O (2020) Aus der Welt. Luchterhand, München
Lesmeister, R (2009) Selbst und Individuation. Brandes & Apsel Verlag, Frankfurt/M
Mattke D, Strauß B, Reddemann L (2009) Keine Angst vor Gruppen. Klett-Cotta, Stuttgart
Nitsun, M (2014) The Anti-Group. Routledge, London
Sloterdijk, P (2009) Du musst Dein Leben ändern. Suhrkamp, Berlin
Smith K K, Berg D N (1988) Paradoxes of Group Life. Jossey-Bass, London
Winnicott, D W (1988) Human nature. Free Association Books, London
Yalom, I (2016) Theorie und Praxis der Gruppenpsychotherapie. Klett-Cotta, Stuttgart

Group Leadership or Group Conducting

13

Abstract

The role of group leadership in group dynamics will be presented in detail. The personal equation of the leaders or conductors plays a significant role. What are their own group experiences? Different attitudes towards the group can massively influence the group process, as we have already seen in Chap. 12. In groups, much unconsciously revolves around the leader, the fantasies about him or her, how they change over time. Important is the "negative capability" (cf. Bion, Attention and Interpretation. Routledge, London, 1984) of the leadership, the ability to establish connections, the belief in what groups have to offer, what they can achieve. However, this also includes that group leaders face their own fear and limitation and exchange ideas with colleagues and continue their professional development.

Without a leader, there is no group. It starts with trained group therapists having to muster the courage to start a group. At this threshold, most (!) group therapists in Germany in the past have so far failed. Only recently, apparently also due to significantly better remuneration and the abolition of the application requirement, things have changed for the better. Not to forget an important remark: Foulkes liked to speak of the group leaders as conductors, since they more lead a group like a conductor leads an orchestra or choir. They have to look what they see and feel, what is played and who performs and cannot control conscious or even unconscious processes in their groups. In some way the group is leading. So in most places I here prefer to use the expression conductor for that reason.

V. Münch, *Group Experience as a Resource*,
https://doi.org/10.1007/978-3-662-70864-4_13

Example

In my work as a psychotherapist, it has happened to me time and again that I met colleagues who either gave up their work as group therapists or never started it. They retreated to the less exhausting, possibly more familiar work of individual therapy. It was difficult to engage in a creative conversation about this, I suspect a lot of discomfort, shame, and frustration as the cause. ◄

13.1 The Connecting Function of the Leaders

As above mentioned Foulkes (e.g. 1974) spoke of the group leader as the conductor, less as the leader. The conductors should not make specifications, not offer authoritarian leadership, as this would block the processes in groups in an unanalytical way. With this, he also wanted to express that leaders should repeatedly facilitate the understanding of group processes by primarily making group interpretations. Unfortunately, this is sometimes not the case in practice, both with Foulkes himself, as the literature shows (see Dalal 1998), and in the author's observation. If one actively expresses understanding for insecurity and temporary regression or disintegration in the group, this can be very helpful. Here I also remember the stabilizing and integrating function of a flash of light, which one of my groups always introduced in such transition phases. Here the participants shortly present their state of mind or can express that they need the time of the group today. The difficulties expressed through tension and contradiction up to devaluation also always have a chance, there are always prospective facets. C. G. Jung (see Vogel 2008) took this up in the concept of finality. As a conductor, I can remind or focus on already achieved progress if it is not conscious. This corresponds to a working method that is not entirely abstinent measured by the classical analytical approach. This approach, also known as "re-framing" from family and systemic therapy, praises participants who show a negative attitude towards the group as courageous, as they also express something for the others. So there really is something positive in the negative!

13.2 The Group-Object-Relation of the Leaders

Nitsun (2014) advocates the thesis that difficult situations that arise in groups can sometimes have their origin in unprocessed parts of the conductors: Possibly a group therapist chooses his job because he himself wants to work on his group issues. Behind constructiveness then lurks hidden devaluation and unconscious aggression. This can lead to patients being included in a group where there would be strong doubts about the meaningfulness of such a step. This particularly affects pronounced narcissistic, but above all antisocial structured personalities with considerable aggression potential. Here, one should not be impressed by the often superficially friendly and adapted persona of the patient and, in case of doubt, protect the group from the strain of such patients. Unprocessed aggressive tendencies of the therapists, including those directed against groups as such, can lead to unconscious identifications with these patients. The unconscious guiding principle would then look something like this: "If the group breaks down, then it didn't deserve any better." Once again, the necessity of including group participants who have enough healthy, normal neurotic parts to be able to work integratively in the sense of group cohesion is reminded. Such patients can also deal more patiently with the difficult patients mentioned, give them more time, and "endure" them, representing the whole group.

The Fit Conductor—Patient

With the influence of the leadership, we enter a very delicate terrain. I advocate the thesis that every group is unconsciously leader-centered, on the one hand, because the participants are consciously selected by them, but on the other hand, and this is the more important point, the various patients can represent certain parts of the therapist's personality. The personal equation must make it possible for the treating person to identify sufficiently with the problems of the patients, in other words, that he or she knows the conflicts at least partially from his or her own perspective, and is touched by the themes and narratives of the patients. Thus, different therapists "get" different patient groups, less guided by diagnosis, but determined in a more subtle, unconscious way by the fit of the respective basic personality.

Another characteristic that sometimes strongly distinguishes groups is that the group processes run differently due to the described patient-therapist fits, both in content and dynamically. There is not *the* exemplary course of a group, similar to individual therapies. Apart from typical insecurities in initial, crisis or final phases, the decisive question is to what extent the leadership can be prevented from projecting its own parts into group participants in such a way that they are misunderstood. The projective identification that is effective in this process can have overall positive and negative effects, in any case, a relationship is established. Sometimes the therapists have to awaken parts of the patients in themselves, i.e., bring in their own (not expressed and preferably conscious), in order to build up genuine interest at all and let the patients benefit from it in this way. Part of this joint process is always somewhat selfish on all sides.

Example

It can be striking how much groups absorb and process the emotions and themes of their group therapists. When I myself was in mourning due to a deathof a relative, I didn't tell my groups about it. Nevertheless, I could observe that the themes of farewell, mourning, and also new beginnings became very dominant in the groups in a more or less direct way. My conclusion was, on the one hand, that unconscious exchange processes had made my situation perceptible to the patients, and on the other hand, I evaluated this phenomenon as an opportunity. When the patients noticed that I myself was dealing with these often difficult emotions, they seized the opportunity and brought in their analogous themes (cf. Frick

2005). This is also an example of the unconscious interplay and a variant of the interaction of social processes in groups.

13.3 The Fears and Hopes of the Group Conductors

Ralf Zwiebel (2018) has dealt extensively with the psychoanalyst's fear of his patients in his books. It is also his merit that we are now able to speak more openly about our own feelings, our subjectivity and its limits and shadow aspects. If I try to create a false image in front of my patients and cannot remain authentic, I can achieve little. And that in the double sense of the word. Therapeutic workers are confronted daily with desires for miracle cures and unrealistic changes shaped by childhood disappointments and frustrations. Therapy largely involves motivating people to deal with what is given and to learn to accept themselves as they are. In the face of this self-acceptance, a change usually begins.

Disappointments are Preprogrammed

It is a truism among therapeutic workers that they have to disappoint those ideas of the patients that are associated with illusory or unrealistic change ideas. For this, they know that patients can benefit from therapy in other, usually still unknown ways. This is especially true for the group: As mentioned, I have experienced that colleagues have decided not to offer group therapy at all because they were hardly able to resist the sometimes angrily articulated demands of their patients. Here we can recognize a danger for therapists: Due to their own high claim to be helpful in a certain way, an identification with the unrealistic expectations of the patients forms. One then gets deeper and deeper into a spiral of justification and self-overexertion. In addition, and here the group comes into play again in the form of the group self (cf. Braun 2016), it is an overexertion to always want to have an overview of all transference and projection levels of the participants. The certainty that the group has self-regulating abilities and also for the good, helps the conductors immensely. Also, a not purely resistance-oriented view of the defense of the participants can contribute to the self-healing powers of each individual configuring. Provided that I believe in the potential that a group can have for the individuals in it.

Example

A younger group participant was initially "mothered" by the group and a lot of patience and understanding was shown for his "youthful escapades". Later, along with his own grown self-confidence, he was also demanded more self-responsibility, for example when it came to behaving responsibly in partnerships. It became clear to him through the reflections of others that he had a strong tendency to self-accusation and self-doubt and only gradually became more confident in recognizing and naming the weaknesses and neuroses of others. It became clear that he had used the milieu of the group for himself to reflect on his emotions and thoughts on the one hand, and to have to control less in his life on the other hand, precisely because of his grown trust in his own impulses and spontaneous decisions. ◂

I can trust that the group participants will deal with themselves and each other in a friendly and binding manner if they have previously internalized the values of the group. Even without complete understanding (this is known to be usually only post-hoc accessible and then only fragmentary) of the complex transference-countertransference processes at a given time, a group is always in a creative process shaped by unconscious and conscious exchange. This trust in what Jung called the ordering, archetypal shape of the self, can help regulate the conductors' fears of the group and its unconscious. She or he rather takes on the role of a witness, a moderator, a catalyst. Archetypically, this is the role of the trickster, the mediator between the areas of consciousness and the unconscious, mythologically represented in the figure of Hermes. In this case of the arrangement of the themes and conflicts by the group, we assume the activity of the "group self". The conductors hopefully know about the creative and destructive forces, with their manifold formations they will have to deal with anew. The process often understood as integration in individual and group therapies is facilitated by the fact that the integration has to be performed beforehand in the analyst, in the form of his assumptions about the contents of the to be integrated and the knowledge about the potential possibility of success.

13.4 Group Therapists Need Groups

The conductors of a group are always also a part of it, they do not exist outside of this group. There is no group without conductors and no conductors without a group. The involvement of the conductor implies that it is sometimes difficult to disengage from the mood and atmosphere in a group. It often takes significantly longer to "step out" of the group circle than it does after an individual session. This is also due to the archetypal force of many traumas and defense mechanisms, which are subliminally linked with strong emotions and multiplied by the number of members.

This involvement also means that the therapists, precisely because they are left alone with their own feelings and questions and also doubts after the group, should belong to further groups in order to be able to relieve and reflect there. We are talking about supervision and intervision groups. Often colleagues have known each other for decades, so there is a very trusting and personal atmosphere that makes it easier to report about the sometimes embarrassing or unsettling events in their own groups. Analytical groups are just as unplannable as individual sessions and they should not be. But this makes every session a tabula rasa and surprising turns can always occur. Another often chosen option is to lead groups together with colleagues. Even more so than in individual therapy, it is significant which social groups the conductor participates in, in which social contexts he or she lives. The rootedness and satisfaction that develops from such positive connectedness nourishes and supports the work, because it helps to reconnect inwardly to people and situations that provide support.

References

Bion, W (1984) Attention and Interpretation. Routledge, London
Braun, C (2016) Die therapeutische Beziehung. Kohlhammer, Stuttgart
Dalal, F (1998) Taking the group seriously. Jessica Kingsley Publishers, London
Foulkes, S (1974) Gruppenanalytische Psychotherapie. Klotz, Neulingen
Frick, E (2005) Sich heilen lassen. Echter, Würzburg
Nitsun, M (2014) The Anti-Group. Routledge, London
Vogel, R T (2008) C. G. Jung für die Praxis. Kohlhammer, Stuttgart
Zwiebel, R (2018) Von der Angst, Psychoanalytiker zu sein. Klett-Cotta, Stuttgart

How Do Groups Work?

14

Abstract

What heals in groups? This question seems even more difficult than the question about the effect of individual therapies, not only at first glance. After all, groups represent a far more complex situation of human contact. They lack many characteristics of the rather distant, artificial situation of the individual setting. We want to investigate what causes change. On which levels does change occur at all? What can one understand by this? Is psychological change possible through a "healing through love", as Freud already noted, or does the integration of shadow aspects and negativity work, which is more reminiscent of Jung? Is it the sharing of common foundations of experience that can promote the desired de-idealization of one's own ideas? And how do intervention paths such as interpretation and amplification stand in this context? Are there other forces that can be effective in groups beyond this?

14.1 Healing through Love?

One might agree with the view already expressed by Freud that "healing is through love," as he wrote in a letter to C.G. Jung in 1906 (cf. Freud and Jung 1974, p. 13). This statement, made over a hundred years ago, is all the more astonishing as Freud, on many other occasions, sought to subject the therapeutic relationship to strict rules, also to prevent a repetition of the derailments that had greatly discredited the still young psychoanalysis. The founding fathers of psychoanalysis, including C.G. Jung, the founder of Analytical Psychology, who began to distance himself from Freud from 1913 onwards (cf. Bair 2005), were able to rely primarily on their self-analysis. However, this made them vulnerable to not sufficiently protecting the therapeutic relationships with their patients. The result

V. Münch, *Group Experience as a Resource*,
https://doi.org/10.1007/978-3-662-70864-4_14

was, for example in the relationship between C.G. Jung and his patient Sabina Spielrein, a later analyst, that behavior occurred that was overbearing and in no way consistent with today's ethical standards.

Strict Analytical Superego and Oversteps

The generation of US-American analysts who followed Freud developed stricter and more rigid rules for treatment than Freud himself, perhaps a consequence of these initial misconducts and boundary violations. However, this probably strengthened the analytical superego above all, prospective analysts subjected themselves to strict moral codes externally, which was legitimized by the desire to secure and improve the quality of treatments. But as would be shown in later decades, this identification with an overly strict ideal formation led to an increase in the frustration of the analysts. As the archives of the German Ethics Association suggest (cf. Schleu 2021), there were and are oversteps or abuses of both a sexual nature and in the form of narcissistic power abuse. What was long too little discussable, Quindeau and Schmidbauer (2017) describe in the sense that it is the holding and mirroring love in psychotherapy that can initiate personal change. However, this form of love has nothing to do with erotic-sexual love, desire.

The Change in the Image of the Subjectivity of Analysts

What was lost from focus in the examination of the mechanisms of psychotherapy was the part of the relationship in an analytical dyad that was not transference-related and distorted, but took place quasi on an equal footing, some also speak of the real relationship. Only the intersubjective turn, initiated by the relational further development of self-psychology and initially mainly based in the USA and England, moved the therapeutic relationship and especially the long-neglected subjectivity of the analyst more into the center of considerations. The associated self-deidealization of the analytical profession and thus the reflection of the shadow aspects of the analytical treatment had massive effects on the self-understanding of most analysts. Within these theoretical currents, voices also increasingly became louder that moved the real relationship more into focus and began to investigate its healing effect. Authors like Knoblauch (2014), Jaenicke (2021), Orange et al. (2015) or also Moeller (cf. Krause-Girth 2007) discussed different, personal aspects of the inevitable psychological involvement of therapists with patients. Concepts, like the long-ostracized description of a "corrective emotional experience" as a therapy goal in today's insurance applications, became "respectable", the real relationship component within the analytical relationship received more attention. Considerations on the dialectic of technique and art in the therapeutic relationship (cf. Lesmeister 2005) made it clear that it was quite impossible to comply with the demand for empathy on the one hand, and on the other hand to largely keep oneself and one's own developmental history, own values, own emotions out of the considerations that could lead to interpretations.

Moeller (cf. Krause-Girth 2007) reintroduced "love" into his considerations on group psychotherapy as early as the 1970s. This was recently pointed out by Stuck (2016), who spoke of it in his "Plea for the Group Thought in Analytical

Psychology". The collectively shared psychological processes in the shared "intermediary" space of the group are crucial. The topics and reactions of the group participants are then understood as just one variation, one manifestation and reflection of these humanity themes and conflicts that affect all more or less. A perspective that helps to refrain from the *exclusive* consideration of individual suffering and to reflect its context conditions as well. Hirblinger (2023) recently published an interesting theoretical work on the multi-layered nature of the subject, which should always be related to societal processes with its problems.

What does the concept of healing through love mean?
The basis of the considerations made here is that the affectively connoted relationship between group participants can freely develop within the space, as it is also given by the group rules. Experience shows, for example, Stuck (2016), that there is a tendency towards approach and sympathy, even if animosities and conflicts occur in parallel. Moeller (see Krause-Girth 2007) emphasizes the aspect of love in the sense of Agape or Caritas (e.g., the love of the group analyst for the whole group). Stuck (2016) concludes in his plea that it is the significance of predominantly good intersubjective experiences that make up the effectiveness of analytical group therapy. The claimed content convergence between Analytical Psychology and the group idea is not self-explanatory: According to Jung, individuality is opposed to the collective idea. Individuation in Analytical Psychology refers to the differentiation of one's own psychological position from the societal and collective. For some time now, there has been an inner Jungian debate on this topic (see Otscheret and Braun 2005). It is noted that individuation does not automatically lead to isolation, but ultimately to a more intense collective context, as the subjectification of the other is needed.

Psychological development of the individual as a product of group experience
The group process and its effect on the development of the individual is examined in great detail: Stuck (2016) speaks of a construction and deconstruction movement taking place at an unconscious level. He says: "In understanding the other, one's own mental position is formed." (Stuck 2016, p. 47). The preliminary conclusion of the authors in the anthology *Self, I and We* (2016) is: Jungian concepts (inner maturation, individuation, access to transcendent, archetypal content) are well compatible with the group experience, in which an exchange of all at an unconscious level is made possible. The image that Analytical Psychology makes of the map of the soul (see Stein 2000) also expands the perspective on groups. It includes the assumption that all those involved in a therapeutic process, i.e., therapist and patient or in a group the participants, can be thought of as unconsciously connected, namely through the assumption of a collective and social unconscious. Foulkes spoke of the "social unconscious" for group psychotherapy and explicitly referred to the ideas of sociologist Norbert Elias. These concepts are being further developed and applied not only in group analysis, but also in so-called Social Dreaming. It is no coincidence that it is apparently mainly group therapeutic concepts that are capable of further developing the idea of "healing through love".

While Freud or Schmidbauer emphasize the idea of empathy, compassion, and patient, devoted work under certain conditions, the idea of how groups function goes even further.

This requires the assumption of common archetypal basic experiences that people can compare with each other in groups. This happens not only on a verbal level, but especially on an implicit, collective, and atmospheric level. The fact that the group participants learn to see themselves in the other in this way, whether in differentiation or identification, creates psychological structure and the firmness that is needed for coping with reality with the formation of an "I".

14.2 Interpretation or Amplification?

Classical psychoanalysis assumed that treatment can be successful if it is possible to identify those unconscious motives and drive derivatives with whose repression a neurotic patient is usually occupied. Their conscious realization leads to insight and thereby the individual gains more freedom over his experience and his scope of action. Where the "Id" has been, the "Ego" should rule. However, according to all experience of the past 120 years of psychoanalysis, this is not always exactly the case with the unconscious. Often important memories elude, there are quite considerable distortion tendencies in the memory work. Narcissistic and other resistances against interpretations, which should contribute to the understanding of the patient about himself, often do not reach their addressee. Several significant theoretical approaches deal with the causes of this (see Kohut 1976; Kernberg 2009). The approach of Analytical Psychology would be to assume that the unconscious is always only partially and always only indirectly accessible. In therapies, it can therefore only be about establishing the best possible access and contact to these layers of personality, without expecting that once something has become conscious, it will remain in consciousness forever. Similar to a searchlight, the searching and judging consciousness only ever throws a beam of light into a certain, selected area, while other things remain in the dark. If the focus of the spotlight changes, other phenomena become apparent, while others fall back into darkness.

The Unconscious as a Resource

Overall, this seems Sisyphean and ultimately means that life is a constant effort towards consciousness. But this is not too tragic at the same time. Because the experience of being able to look at something previously unconscious, like through a dream, and letting it affect you, often without being able to be explicitly put into words, has a lasting effect. This is particularly evident in treatments that offer creative and imaginative methods in combination with analytical psychotherapy (e.g., sandplay therapy, active imagination, subjective-level dream analysis). Some of these methods can also be applied in a group context. In Analytical Psychology, it is assumed that the unconscious is not only generated from repressed content and emotions, but represents a *resource* that is capable of providing images and also solutions if one directs attention to it. This is, of course, a different perspective than that of classical revealing psychoanalysis.

Unfolding and Jointly Witnessing Unconscious Processes
My experience as an individual and group therapist, but also my own self-experience and many contacts with colleagues and friends suggest that the quiet joint experience and viewing of what is, is effectively transformative. Much has been written about what this process looks like in detail and how one can imagine these transformation processes. For example, Winfred Bion (1997) speaks of "Faith in O", Christopher Bollas of the transformation object, to conceptualize transformation processes. In the sense of Bollas (2011), a group would be a "multidimensional transformative object". Transformation is not a self-runner in psychotherapies: Unfortunately, I personally know people who have undergone partly years, if not decades, of rather classically oriented psychoanalyses, and who still have great difficulties in beneficially implementing what they have experienced and learned about themselves in everyday life and coping with life. This may be due to an insight that has remained too cognitive, an insufficiently deep bonding experience in the treatment, and also the structural inability to allow certain affects to approach oneself. Nevertheless, the multitude of such "cases" gives rise to doubts as to whether psychological changes can be brought about solely by means of "insight" and "interpretation". The question is rather, at least since the so-called intersubjective turn, which goes back to theoretical influences from the Anglo-American sphere, whether the influence of the real encounter and a corrective emotional experience gained there with a resonant counterpart and overall the hitherto unknown mental "set" of the therapists has contributed to the fact that significant changes are emerging.

The Changed Handling of Interpretations
The more warlike metaphorics of early theory formation, which showed itself in the language of interpretation, has greatly regressed. It was recognized that especially narcissistically structured patients or borderliners can feel very attacked by defensive interpretations and thus resistance was rather reinforced. Nowadays, many structural disorders are successfully treated in groups, also with psychodynamic approaches, but in many cases with DBT. It also depends on what definition of interpretation one has. All in all, it can be stated today that interpretations are given less significance for various reasons (cf. Jaenicke 2021). Biographical and thus saturated interpretations are receding in favor of "unsaturated", more open interpretations (cf. Will 2016). Many group authors are more concerned with connecting, re-framing, (perhaps amplifying?) and integrating. It is known today: Interpretations in groups can also trigger "anti-group behavior". For example, envy of the (all-knowing?) leaders and hatred because of the content of the interpretations are aroused. Group interpretations, if they are more comprehensive and understanding, can on the other hand be integratively effective. Nitsun (2014) reports an example in which he linked the group's undisciplined, careless handling of rules and the framework and thus with each other with the behavior of

the participants' parents, thus revealing an unconscious identification of the group participants with their careless parents.

Example

A participant in his late 30s initially presented a strong entanglement in his relationship. He seemed very eager to connect with his partner, who, however, responded little. A repetition of the disappointing relationship with his depressive mother became apparent. After some time, more conflictual feelings towards the conductor emerged. Without these conflicts and relationship constellations being extensively interpreted biographically, the patient developed internally. Apparently, he benefited from the open, non-judgmental, accepting listening and communication in the group. After a longer period, he decided to end the relationship, not without inner struggles and feelings of guilt. The relationship with the conductor and other men in the group also relaxed. One must assume an internal triangulation that the patient was able to carry out in the group through the group, because on the one hand the close identification with the mother was loosened, on the other hand the oedipal rivalry with the father was re-enacted and made identifiable. Neither the repetition of the mother relationship in the partnership nor the character of the rivalry with the group conductor were explicitly addressed by the group or the leader. All of this shows how sensible it is to assume a self or a group self that sets development in motion. Through the new experience of a compassionate, friendly confrontation and reciprocal exchange in the group, which expands or corrects internal assumptions, mental structures undergo a change. The patient's personality appeared more integrated and mature, he led his life more actively and reflectively than before, changed situations in his professional and private life that were unsuitable for him, developed new creative interests, and also found a new partner. and finally married. ◄

Schmidbauer (2023) also reports good experiences with amplifying interventions, especially with narcissistically toned problems. He speaks of "chatting", the seemingly harmless conversation that one should be able to engage in, because here the (mostly male) patient does not sense any overpowering and above all no humiliation, here he predominantly experiences himself as the master of events. One comes, as I understand Schmidbauer, through the back door, "normalizes" his patients through the seemingly normal conversation. The prerequisite for this is that one engages with the patient's defenses and also temporarily suspends one's own therapeutic superego.

14.3 How Does Change Happen?

To enable development, it requires (speaking with Jung) the capture of shadow aspects, also an awareness of the "Anti-Group" (cf. Sect. 12.2). If this is recognized, there are better chances that a group will develop autonomously and self-regulatively. The idea for the potential for change lies hidden in Foulkes's conception of the matrix: Here many lives, and through them culture, their history and mythology meet, as well as past, present and future. This is the transpersonal potency of the matrix. But how can aggression (especially hate) be held and transformed in such a way that it leads to beneficial, integrative and not destructive developments overall? Nitsun (2014) believes that the "disturbance" caused by Anti-Group impulses can lead to dissolution, but also to temporary deregulation, after which new structures can be built that are more resilient and integrated than before. For him, it is always about an interplay of destructive and constructive forces. Too great an idealized one-sidedness, on the other hand, could ultimately lead to totalitarian conditions.

Example

Three different group participants are confronted one after the other with their behavior and impact on others in a group: It is very difficult for the others to follow their often expansive and detailed narratives and reports. Even for the conductor, very little is often perceptible for a long time and listening is strenuous, evoking rather aversive feelings. The group participants initially react, as usual, patiently. If such a situation accumulates, there is always someone who eventually loses patience and confronts with a stronger affect: that it is difficult to follow the narrative, what it is actually about and whether the others also feel that they perceive little to nothing. It is very important for those addressed or criticized that the group does this on the basis of warm interest in their group member. The choice of words is very important due to the high risk of humiliation of the rather narcissistic co-patients in this case. The criticism often initially triggers surprise and indeed anger. One feels interrupted, disturbed, not understood. But this anger of the original narrators is essential, because it is the actual affect that was repressed, which led to the narrative being experienced as so colorless. The group members are actually only demanding what is already constellated in the unconscious of the person concerned. If those addressed now become angry in turn, a confrontation follows, which is ideally resolved by recognizing the affect as their own. ◀

Often, these patients are reserved and passive in their self-perception, but are perceived by others as dominant and controlling. It can be very enlightening when someone gains access to these aspects and affects, previously only perceived by others in the group. This can explain why these individuals repeatedly encounter situations of rejection in their lives outside the group, or even unconsciously create such situations, leading to cumulative frustrations. Experiencing this under different conditions in the group and achieving a different outcome and contact with others can be very illuminating and relieving. Although initially, these are difficult feelings to bear that become conscious, need to be endured, and must find expression.

The Complexity Theory and Change Processes in Groups
Stuck (2020) has vividly demonstrated for analytical group therapy how the change processes in complex processing in the group look in detail. He shows that in the group process, a transformation of the complexly charged behavior of the participants away from rather rigid, restricted behaviors, away from the "elementary character" of the archetypically shaped complex and towards its "transformation character" (cf. Neumann 1994) takes place. Change can occur when the frightening aspects, for example, of a negative mother or father complex, can gradually be perceived as less frightening through personal encounters in the group. Because the complex events in a group also affect other participants, there is an unconscious and then increasingly conscious exchange about this topic. This has a transformative effect as it makes the topic concrete and reveals it in its many facets. The experience of the ubiquity of complexes can also be deeply touching and transformative (cf. Stuck 2020). Stuck also mentions that in groups, there is usually a desire for the transformation character of the mother complex. It is therefore about the experience of positively and development-promoting properties of the psychotherapy group perceived as a mother figure. The mobilization of inner forces that can promote the change of group participants is part of the functioning of groups. However, these forces are archetypically composed and therefore must be transformed by the group in its process into internally understandable and empathetic experiences. Remaining in the elementary character due to traumatic, frightening experiences can hinder the process of unfolding and emancipation of the personality. Stuck (2020) thus concludes that it is primarily the healing effect of (genuine) relationships that are effective in groups.

14.4 Theoretical Aspects of Transformation

There are many considerations regarding the mode of action of analytical psychotherapy and specifically the mode of action of analytical group psychotherapy. Especially in connection with the last example of long-winded, annoying storytelling that evokes aversive feelings, it is important to experience that the group and the therapists "survive" the (fantasized) and expressed aggression (cf. Winnicott 1960, 1974). The group "survives": it continues and this strengthens the participants' confidence that they too can withstand life with their affects. In other words: The group can thus gain the experience that it contains and can withstand or "survive" destructive impulses, and this strengthens the constructive psychological parts of the individuals as well. The group metabolizes the difficult affects, so to speak. This can lead to mourning processes and genuine concern for others.

Groups can also be seen as a transitional object in the Winnicottian sense, as the conductors as providers of security are gradually replaced by the group itself. Nitsun concludes that Foulkes' theory overestimates the importance of what stands between people: differences, separation, social gap, ignorance, other barriers. In principle, Nitsun says, it is good to approach group work with Foulkes' "act of faith", but one should not be naive.

The Social Animal

More recent, popular scientific works like those by Brooks (2011) have elaborated for a larger audience that we indeed have a lot in common on deeper levels, which can explain the functioning of groups. Brooks assumes different layers of information under whose influence our behavior stands. The longer the influence of our evolutionary past lasts, the more sustainable is the imprinting by its form and content. These influencing factors are all located between genetics and upbringing (cf. Brooks 2011). He thus assumes a layered model of the instances of the human psyche that also control our group behavior.

The background of the current group experience is always the early deficient experience regarding a holding environment of the participants. An attack on the group always has a defensive character. It is intended to prevent the participants from taking personal responsibility for their difficulties and accepting the pain of learning and psychological growth. This happens in many gradations. The task of the conductors is to educate about this process of defense, but also to make the underlying emotional situation understandable and acceptable.

14.5 The Successful Group Process

With the growing together of a group and many shared experiences, there is usually an increased tolerance for ambiguity, but fears of the departure of individuals can trigger regressive processes again. Each group develops its own history, which the participants are quite proud of. They see themselves as part of the narration that only arises through their own participation in the group. The individual group members experience the group as a given "added value". The group is the group and not the sum of its participants. It develops its own identity. Group therapists who lead several groups can describe this well. The different groups sometimes also give themselves symbolically understandable "names" and their own narration (cf. Braun 2016).

Especially slow-open groups with their recurring farewells can also trigger early fears of abandonment. However, in my experience, a group acquires a steadily more stable ability to deal with this, whether it is planned departures or sudden breaks, which of course shake the group more. The slow-open characteristic of the group itself becomes a symbol for change and has an effect on the participants. It challenges them to constructively face changes in the group, and thus analogously in the course of life. The effect that the participants are thrown back more onto themselves and their (also common) resources with the farewells has a double consequence: it can lead to wishes for regression, but also to progression. It becomes clear here that "Anti-Group" can have therapeutic effects and can ultimately prove to be helpful. Nitsun (2014) also reminds us of the dynamics of depressive and paranoid-schizoid position and the oscillation between these positions conceived by Klein as helpful.

The Group "Dreams"
The group process as an unfolding unconscious process can also be compared to the experience of the unconscious, as it tends to present itself through the realization of dreams. If one perceives the manifest group process from this perspective as the unfolding of latent unconscious thoughts, the course of group sessions resembles the course of individual dreams. This is particularly often evident in the situation when someone new is admitted to the group. The other group participants quickly grasp the possibilities and defense formations of the newcomer and often react extraordinarily empathetically and clearly. How one can imagine this process in detail and what advantages such a perspective can have for the group conductor and the group itself, the author has tried to describe in his contribution in the book of Claus Braun *Dream Work in Groups* (Münch 2022). The basic idea is again that the unconscious of the group as a self-regulating system determines the course and the topics of the togetherness and that one can confidently surrender to this process, while trying to observe it attentively as a conductor.

14.5.1 Overcoming the Fear of the Unknown

Crucial for the successful group process is that the fear of the unknown and the strangers is gradually reduced. Strangers become familiar and sometimes almost friendly relationships develop, even if these find a different expression in group psychotherapy than in life "outside". Since group psychotherapy confronts with much more real strangers and unknowns than individual psychotherapy, it understandably also initially causes more fear. This applies to patients, but also to the therapists themselves. Analytical groups with their unstructuredness and openness frustrate dependency needs from the start, leading to fear and confusion. Hence the often great resistance to giving up the individual setting. Groups span the polarity generally valid in the therapeutic situation between the former childlike and the current adult position. And this in a very complex way. The complexity of the communicative levels in a group is at the same time an advantage, as fixations, one-sidedness and premature projections can be resolved more quickly. In addition, a group challenges the ability to really deal with the otherness of others. Beyond the image projected by me, there is a real other with his individual history and his own defense. Difference and participation are in a reciprocal relationship. Fantasies are under much greater pressure to measure up to reality. A group offers a complex experience. The complexity of the processes, which are hardly ever to be overlooked, is strenuous to follow, but always exciting. There is the real level, the transference level, the level of projections, the primordial level of the collective unconscious.

Groups thus reactivate intrapsychic *and* interpersonal tensions. This involves the difficult topics and affects of competition, rivalry, envy, dominance, submission, criticism, rejection, group pressure, scapegoats and hostility. And it can be stated that groups usually oscillate between development, standstill and regression. Without the positive forces that groups also release, their mode of operation would hardly be explainable. According to Nitsun (2014), these include joy, creativity, participation, insight, wisdom, but also beauty and aesthetics.

14.5.2 The Archetypal Level

Through the deep inner connection that the individual has with the surrounding collective, and because this connection is strongly triggered by the coming together of a group, one can interpret individual suffering as the suffering of the collective. Group therapists who see the group as a psychological unit thus ask what the suffering of a part of the group says about the whole group. Accordingly, group conflicts always first become visible in conflicts of individuals. The psychology of Erich Neumann, which has dealt extensively with the level of collective development of individuals, can contribute much here (see Neumann 2004). To investigate how group analysis and collective, archetypal development can theoretically be linked is a promising future field of research. The group forum within the professional society DGAP (German Society for Analytical Psychology) has recently dealt with this question.

The development of individuals in and with a group is possible because all are connected to the same group-related archetype. The connection to the collective dimension of one's own unconscious refers to this always already mentally-spiritually being related to others. In this respect, a successful group process always enables an approach to these experiential dimensions inherent in being human, as they present themselves in individual fates. From here it is not far to the assumption of the archetypal psychology of James Hillman (see Hillman 2004), who spoke of the fact that in therapies it is primarily about allowing experiences and witnessing them together. This often brings about profound psychological change.

The Negativity of Mental Events

For Giegerich (2020, 2021), what is therapeutically effective is to be considered a mental event that cannot be captured in terms of individual psychology. With negativity, Giegerich describes the eventful and unpredictable in therapeutic transformation processes, the processes are not solely provable in a positivist way. What is capable of changing individuals in a group is not solely due to the personal unconscious, the interactions, the transference and countertransference reactions, nor the culture prevailing in the group and the language regulations or the atmosphere prevailing in it. Mental change happens quasi en passant, without initially detectable cause, with surprising twists and turns and ultimately unfathomable. However, respect for these processes is paradoxically the prerequisite for their effectiveness. Any hasty classification or attempt to control and standardize processes would be counteracted by the mental, according to Giegerich. His way of thinking can be very helpful in preventing adherence to concretisms, such as rigid subject-object or cause-effect thinking, or a false pathologization. The archetypal, the mental in the narrower sense, as Giegerich views it, is always present as an unknown third from the beginning, be it in a dyadic or a group situation.

Example

Every group becomes a witness to the constellating unconscious themes and the overlap of personal and group themes in its course. In my experience, this creates a greater distance to the hitherto virulent, neurotic mechanisms. Stagings, in which a desire for contact seems to be effective, but also its defense, reduce. This suggests less fear and overall more familiarity and serenity. Fear and also negativity, hatred and destruction have less impact on the group process when they can increasingly be recognized. Through the individual interaction sequences, manifest themes are discussed on the surface, but subliminally it is about more general aspects of human coexistence affecting the whole group. In a slightly altered form, this already becomes visible when the group works on a topic of a group member and asks what dynamics are "behind it". The classification of the everyday into transpersonal, psychic dynamics affecting all participants is important for reducing complexity and helps in the development of better affect and self-regulation. In this way, the individuals and the group develop simultaneously. ◀

14.5.2.1 The Dissociability of the Psyche

Referring to the model of Jungian "dissociability of the psyche", which can exist not only in a pathological state, the group setting opens a number of interesting points of connection. Jung (1973), despite his group-critical attitude, recognized: "The self, the actual center of the individual, is by its nature a plurality. It is, so to speak, a group. It represents a collectivity and creates groups when it acts in a positive sense." (cf. Jung 1973, p. 130 f.). If the goal in Analytical Psychology is to bring previously insufficiently connected, too far dissociated part psyches or complexes into relationship with each other, then a group could offer the psyche the opportunity to project previously unconnected inner psychic parts onto different participants. This would initially be associated with greater visibility of the complexes within the overall dynamics of the group. The psyche of the individuals would thus also be given the opportunity to reintroject the projected own parts identificatorically. Or processes in the sense of Bion's container-contained could be assumed. If the group, the group self symbolically and thus projective-identificatory stands for the whole of the respective individual psyche, then this can interpret the diversity experienced in the group as an indication of its own diversity within its wholeness. The disassembly of previously disparate experiences and feelings can bring inner insight and a broadening of perspective on oneself. This creates self-distance, reflection and increasing awareness. The inner is reflected, so to speak, in the interactive field of the group and could then be reintegrated and used for psychic growth.

14.5.2.2 The Effect of the Group Self in Analytical Psychology

Braun (2016) summarizes what, in his estimation, works in analytical groups. The individuals in a therapeutic group become part of the group matrix and also of the transpersonally conceived group self to varying degrees. In the best case, a part of one's own identity is given up in favor of the others and the group, which also makes projections and transferences more bearable. The analyst must also open themselves to these processes. The sense of "we" that arises in groups with a positive course helps to tolerate difficult behavior of individual patients. Even the "self-becoming" of the group, if it once demarcates itself from the group leadership, is in principle an emancipatory signal! The term "group self" to my knowledge goes back to Erich Neumann (2004), who describes the effect of groups as an "external self". Here, members experience a group as if it had its own consciousness, unconsciousness, and its own possibilities for action. Thus, groups are "self-regulating treatment systems" (cf. Braun 2016, pp. 89–90). Essential for their culture in the therapeutic area, where it is about respect, honesty, tolerance, flexibility, is the influence of the conductors. These values are usually implicitly represented in the therapeutic attitude (cf. Münch 2021).

Summary

With Braun (2016), I would like to summarize the current view of Analytical Psychology on groups in advance (cf. Chap. 15): There is a "double and archetypal structuring and development process that takes place in every group, provided it is allowed to unfold as a self-regulating treatment system. A dynamic matrix is created as a transitional space in which an emergent and final oriented transpersonal subject, the group self, can express itself." (Braun 2016, p. 90). This view contrasts decidedly with the psychoanalytic view of groups. One could also say that the effect of groups from this perspective is due to the emergence of a "swarm intelligence" that tries to overcome resistance and defense phenomena. This is possible and here the convergence of Jungian thinking and phenomena observable in groups is shown, if one considers the unconscious as a resource and as a "treasure" in which solutions are hidden that can be made visible and effective through and in groups.

References

Bair, D (2005) C. G. Jung – eine Biografie. Knaus, München

Bion, W R (1997) Transformationen. Suhrkamp, Frankfurt/M

Bollas, C (2011) The Christopher Bollas Reader. Routledge, London

Braun, C (2016) Gruppenselbst und Gruppenmatrix. In: Schimkus M, Stuck U (Eds.) Selbst, Ich und Wir. Brandes & Apsel Verlag, Frankfurt/M

Braun, C (2022) (Hrsg.) Traumarbeit in Gruppen. Brandes & Apsel Verlag, Frankfurt/M

Britten, U, Quindeau, I, Wolfgang Schmidbauer, W (2017) Der Wunsch nach Nähe – Liebe und Begehren in der Psychotherapie. Verlag Vandenhoeck und Ruprecht, Göttingen

Brooks, D (2011) The Social Animal. Short Books, London

Freud, S, Jung, C G (1974) Briefwechsel. Hrsg.: McGuire, W, Sauerländer, W. Fischer, Frankfurt/M
Giegerich, W (2020) What is Soul? Routledge, London
Giegerich, W (2021) Coniunctio. Dusk Owl Books, London
Hillman, J (2004) Archetypal Psychology. Spring Publications, Thompson
Hirblinger, A (2023) Über Tabus im psychoanalytischen Dialog und das Gebot des Einbezugs gesellschaftlicher Realitäten als Quelle psychischen Leidens. In: Ztschr Forum für Psychoanalyse, Heft 3/2023, Springer, Heidelberg
Jaenicke, C (2021) Das Risiko der Verbundenheit. Psychosozial-Verlag, Gießen
Jung, C G (1973) Briefe in drei Bänden. Walter, Olten
Kernberg, O (2009) Borderline-Störungen und pathologischer Narzissmus. Suhrkamp, Frankfurt/M
Knoblauch, S H (2014) The Musical Edge of Therapeutical Dialogue. Routledge, London
Kohut, H (1976) Narzissmus. Suhrkamp, Frankfurt/M
Krause-Girth, C (Hrsg) (2007) Die Gruppe, das Paar und die Liebe: Zum Wirken von Michael Lukas Moeller. Psychosozial-Verlag, Gießen
Lesmeister, R (2005) Technik und Beziehung. In: Otscheret L, Braun C (Hrsg) Im Dialog mit dem Anderen. Brandes & Apsel Verlag, Frankfurt/M
Münch, V (2021) Die therapeutische Haltung. Kohlhammer, Stuttgart
Münch, V (2022) Das Gruppenselbst träumt. In: Braun, C (Eds.) Traumarbeit in Gruppen. Brandes & Apsel Verlag, Frankfurt/M
Neumann, E (2004) Ursprungsgeschichte des Bewusstseins. Patmos, Ostfildern
Neumann, E (1994) Die große Mutter. Walter, Düsseldorf
Nitsun, M (2014) The Anti-Group. Routledge, London
Orange, D et al. (2015) Intersubjektivität in der Psychoanalyse. Brandes & Apsel Verlag, Frankfurt/M
Otscheret L, Braun C (2005) Im Dialog mit dem Anderen. Brandes & Apsel Verlag, Frankfurt/M
Schleu, A (2021) Umgang mit Grenzverletzungen. Professionelle Standards und ethische Fragen in der Psychotherapie. Springer, Heidelberg
Schmidbauer, W (2023) https://wolfgang-schmidbauer.de/3753/das-verhaeltnis-von-deutung-und-amplifikation. Stand: 22.09.2023
Stein, M B (2000) C. G. Jungs Landkarte der Seele. Walter, Düsseldorf
Stuck, U (2016) Plädoyer für den Gruppengedanken in der Analytischen Psychologie. In: Schimkus M, Stuck U (Eds.) Selbst, Ich und Wir. Brandes & Apsel Verlag, Frankfurt/M
Stuck, U (2020) Analytische Gruppentherapie: Komplexbearbeitung in der Gruppe.- Die heilende Wirkung von Beziehung in Gruppen. In: Pröstler M, Mattke, D (Hrsg) Formen ambulanter Gruppentherapie. Springer, Heidelberg
Will, H (2016) Ungesättigte und gesättigte Deutungen. Psyche, 1/2016, S 2–23. Klett-Cotta, Stuttgart
Winnicott, D W (1960) The theory of the parent-infant relationship. International Journal of Psychoanalysis, 41: 585–595
Winnicott, D W (1974) Ichverzerrung in Form des wahren und des falschen Selbst. In: Reifungsprozesse und fördernde Umwelt. S. Fischer, Frankfurt/M, 182–199

The Group in Analytical Psychology 15

Abstract

Only in recent years have the German Society for Analytical Psychology and group analysts working within it dealt in depth with the question of how Jungian psychoanalysis and its sometimes long-standing group practice can be conceptually thought together. From this initiative, several symposia, a congress, many articles, and several joint books have emerged so far. It became clear that the well-known concepts of group analysis, such as that of Foulkes, but also the psychology of Erich Neumann, are quite compatible with modern group analytical concepts. Further activities are being planned.

15.1 Farewell to Purely Introverted Individuation

C. G. Jung (1995) pursued the idea that self-realization, the process of individuation, generally speaking the development and maturation of the personality, could be achieved primarily through the description of the internal processes involved in the associated transformation. For this purpose, he used the systematic approach of the symbol system of alchemy, which he elaborated in 1946 for psychotherapeutic practice, which in his view had already unconsciously attempted to capture these internal processes in linguistic images. The image of the common bath, into which the two participants of an encounter step (an image also for the therapeutic encounter), to emerge changed from it, however, already contains the idea that personal further development requires the encounter with a real other in addition to contact with the mediating third party (the bath). Inner change processes are triggered by these encounters, such as by getting to know an important person, or also by starting therapy.

V. Münch, *Group Experience as a Resource*,
https://doi.org/10.1007/978-3-662-70864-4_15

With the theory of intersubjectivity, a paradigm shift has occurred in psychoanalysis over the past 30 years. To a much greater extent than was previously the case, a place is given to the other, including the real other, the subjectivity of analysts, for example. Development is seen as an event that arises in relationships and through bonds. This is important and correct. And yet, the focus on the dyadic two-person relationship overlooks the fact that we are all woven into complex relationship networks, i.e., groups, and derive our stability and identity from them. In the group context, unconscious exchange and communication gain an almost insurmountable complexity. Everything we feel and think is related to the world in which we grow up and live. This applies to the time when we are shaped and our emotional landscape is emerging, and also to the present time when we can possibly make corrective experiences in psychotherapy.

Example

I have repeatedly encountered patients who were able to benefit from analytical individual therapy, but who continued to complain about feelings of being cut off, of inner isolation. When I then admitted them to a group, I began to understand better why this might be the case. Their behavior was remarkable compared to that of many others. They tried to control the group rather than really getting involved in the flow of events. All in all, they seemed more tense, more strained, the group seemed to trigger great fear in them. Many tried to understand what was going on, primarily intellectually. Sometimes this seemed bizarre and incomprehensible, as much of the obvious was not perceived, expressed, and probably not thought by them. Their comments on the problems of others sometimes seemed inappropriate and forced, somehow "thought around the corner" and affectively rather impoverished. These people vividly and painfully show their distress, as one experiences how much the perceived inner non-belonging to groups makes life difficult and without perspective. The transformative power of a group, on the other hand, can bring people to themselves. It can lead to learning to see oneself more realistically, more appropriately, perhaps even more kindly in the face of others. However, there is also that archetypal fear of being absorbed in groups, which makes an uninhibited, open being in groups very difficult for these people. This is due to the difficult object experiences that these patients have internalized. ◄

Since we humans are always placed in social contexts and origins and also represent them, therapeutic small groups are always a downsized version of what is happening in society (cf. Dalal 1998). Certainly, individuals meet here, but if one considers that there are many overlaps due to similar socialization rituals, class-specific codes and habits, which are also expressed linguistically, then one already has a clue as to what could become bindingly effective in such groups. This actual or presumed similarity of individuals is also taken into account when compiling according to the Noah's Ark principle (Yalom 2016): Relief is provided by admitting at least two participants with similar personality structures, also disease backgrounds, so that identification possibilities exist, especially at the beginning. The small group as a micro-laboratory of society allows people to feel their commonality, also their culturally determined commonality. Yalom (2016) also speaks of the universality of suffering, which can be recognized and acknowledged. After all, the culture of psychotherapy is added to the previous experiences with its perspectives, concepts and sometimes greatly simplified ideas by laypeople. Eva Illouz (2009) has taken a detailed and critical position on the shaping of Western societies by this psychological perspective that permeates many subcultures.

The Influence of Group Culture
If we do not primarily imagine people living in dyadic relationships, but always embedded in groups that have diverse intersections, sometimes overlapping each other on different levels, then this influence also applies to the therapy group: The prevailing culture in a group becomes what most sustainably shapes the people in it. The unspoken part of a group, represented by the values and behavior of the conductors and the way of thinking about oneself, others, and the world that is implemented with it, indirectly shapes the group process. Again and again, groups then engage in cyclical disputes with tendencies of devaluation, disappointment, and aggression. It often bitterly backfires when destructive tendencies are not recognized, named, and a way of dealing with them can be found.

From what has been said so far, one could explain why it is sometimes easier in groups to dissuade people from the destructive imprinting by their primary groups, at least to an extent that a developmental process can be resumed. When it comes to this, the attachment to the person of the psychoanalysts sometimes appears to be too weak. The destructive, sometimes even sadomasochistic, social relationships of the patients outside the practice have such a persistence and pull that patients often fail to achieve the internal detachment process, which, given the transference, also always means the detachment process from the therapists, on their own. The entire group of origin, i.e., the family, the peers, the sickening environment, often with people who show a clear structural similarity to the pathology of the parents, a whole group of real and internalized others keeps the patients firmly in the compulsions to repeat, brooding, and self-doubts. A whole group together with the therapists already represents a certain counterforce.

15.2 Once Again: The Level of Archetypes

Brigitte Dorst (2016) has highlighted the importance of the archetypal level of psychic life in working with groups. In her work *The Archetype of the Group*, Dorst speaks of the elements that could underlie the work and thus also the effectiveness in the group on a deeper level than the interpersonal-communicative. According to Jungian terminology, she uses different terms than psychoanalytic group psychotherapists. Above all, the experience of the group as a self-symbol is in the foreground in this view (cf. Sect. 14.5.2). Through the work on archetypal relationship patterns, roles, and group situations, the processing of complex constellations, dealing with shadow projections, beyond the persona, the group experience could, according to Dorst, contribute to a greater sense of meaning, an experience of the greater whole, which is healing in itself. A group process is thus both a differentiation and integration process at the same time. Being different and being the same becomes simultaneously tangible.

From my point of view, this applies to the description of those processes that can neither be explained solely from the biographical-personal nor from the interpersonal conflict dynamics in the group. Archetype and archetypal as fundamental, formative structural features of our psyche show themselves, for example, in the "energetic charge" of group dynamics, in the tension of opposites between the always positive *and* negative aspects of the archetype, in symbols and images from the collective unconscious, in the creative process of the group as well as the transformation and healing potential of the numinosity of the group phenomenon itself (cf. Dorst 2016).

Example

It is fascinating to observe the changing handling of aggressive impulses in groups. While at the beginning mainly aggressive feelings from the external relationships are reported, usually a phase of aggressive fantasies about the group leaders follows. Ironically, they can also be accused of dealing too little with the topic of "aggression". Only after building greater trust in the stability of the relationships within the group do participants dare to criticize each other and express their displeasure. This in turn provides relief, as the feared disintegration processes do not occur. On the contrary: usually, the group grows together more in this way. ◄

The Convergence of Topics

Throughout each group process, it can be observed that the topics of the participants increasingly converge. Everyone realizes that there are typical conflict situations of mental life that affect several, if not all, participants. The reciprocity of contributions usually also increases significantly the longer a group exists. A recently started group noted at the end of about the tenth joint session that they had extensively discussed the topic "relationship to mothers" for the first time. This involved several patients having difficulties in setting boundaries against possessive and complaining mothers. This was noted as a common topic and noticeably increased the group's sense of identity and coherence. The typical conflict constellations or fundamental topics such as the archetypal mother, father, and triangulation topics can each be assigned to a complex event, which means that it involves the activation of psychological areas that are affectively charged in a characteristic way (for example, mother complex, authority complex, inferiority complex).

A common topic initially is the accusations against the parents for not having treated their children, i.e., the patients, well enough. Especially at the beginning of group processes, these boundary movements are very widespread and also very important. This ultimately serves to establish group coherence. Soon a group realizes, and this more so the longer it lasts and already has participants who have been there for a longer time, that the affects do not serve a purpose in themselves and that it is also about using aggression sensibly and constructively for one's own development, instead of constantly working off the previous generation.

What is the Nature of Relationships in Groups?

To initiate these processes, Dorst emphasizes that it requires the willingness of group therapists for real encounters (Buber's I-Thou). This corresponds to her demand for the practice of intersubjective psychoanalysis, as it was vividly demonstrated for Analytical Psychology by Otscheret (2005) or Lesmeister (2009). This perspective implies that the therapists, on the one hand, move in a role, but on the other hand, also reveal themselves as human beings (cf. Münch 2021). Yalom (2005, 2016) also presents himself as a storyteller in both his professional books and his novels. This includes targeted self-disclosure at times. If patients, after a certain duration of treatment, are able to reduce their transference tendency, the therapists can also become more noticeable and visible in their limitation, in their experience as human beings. This can have healing effects. If the person of the therapist no longer needs to be idealized, but is rather met with gratitude and respect, this is a sign that the self-ideal has moved away from the narcissistic pole on the patient's side.

Example

After I had a dispute with a patient of a group in a one-on-one conversation, she complained about me at the next group meeting to the others. Some of the group reacted remarkably: They tried to calm the fellow patient and convey to her that she should be happy to be part of the group, and that she is not so dependent on me (which of course represented both hubris and aggression in addition to the real aspects). But it was also a statement of the group about its own self-understanding, which thus declared and showed that it understood itself as its own force and granted itself a certain independence. ◂

For Dorst (2016), it is the numinous, fascinating, and hard-to-name quality of the group that has healing efficacy: The group is experienced as a place of change, transformation, rediscovery of unconscious parts, letting go of constricting persona masks, invigoration of ego forces, and centering on the self (cf. Dorst 2016). The process is influenced by conscious and unconscious personal and collective components. The archetype of the group appears when people communicate with each other in a common social space. This process is consciously-unconsciously based on essential existential basic assumptions in groups. Analogous to the individual psyche, the collective experience level of the individuals contained in it with groups manifests itself in groups. This elevates the group to the level of a symbol in which psychic forces are represented. Thus, the group can symbolically be perceived as a good place, chaos, devouring or also good mother, and much more. Group myths can also develop. Jung meant that therapy means finding one's own myth, asking oneself the question: "How am I meant?" This question can also be asked by a group.

The Influence of Group Leadership

The intervention styles of group therapists naturally correspond with these unconscious, archetypal images of the group. The influence of the therapist's personality is repeatedly emphasized by group analysts. What applies to individual treatment applies even more to the group. This also results from the much greater transparency of the therapists. They are much more "under observation" due to the comparisons and perspectives from the group members. In the transference, rejected behaviors can be identified as well as characteristics that invite model learning. Identification usually occurs with a changed, more open and accepting approach to one's own self and one's own problems. These are recognized as universally human and can be better accepted, as one no longer feels so alone with them. As a result, they lose their potency, as the individual no longer has to deal with rejecting or wanting to get rid of problematic aspects of themselves. This desire to "get rid of" often determines many in their therapy motivation, until they realize that it is about unavoidable human feelings and conflicts that only become unbearable when one tries to banish them from one's life, because there is no one who could relieve them. Behind this often lies the wishful thinking of a problem-free and conflict-free life, which is often conveyed as an ideal in culture.

The Multiplicity of Perspectives and Processes

If one summarizes the considerations of the original contributions of Analytical Psychology to group theory and therapy, then the group is for them the place where individuals can simultaneously experience individuality and connection with others. The group helps by reminding of the existence of a personal "self" that also encompasses the collective dimension through the activation and experience of the group self. This has a centering, calming, and structuring effect on the individual group members, but in turn on the group as a whole. However, this is only possible when the initial "group illusion", which includes exaggerated expectations of the leaders as well as a "group narcissism", i.e., an overemphasis on one's own group, could largely be overcome. Stuck speaks of a "transitional phase" (Stuck 2016, p. 74), after which one should not imagine a psychotherapeutic group as a force characterized primarily by regressive processes. Thus, a successful group process does not contradict the individuation of the individual, as Jung himself critically pointed out. Stuck quotes Claus Braun (2003), who says about the development of the (Jungian understood) self that it "does not remain dyadic, it must become triadic, perhaps even multiple on a mature level" (quoted according to Stuck, 2016, p. 74). This also corresponds to the sociological perspective as developed by Vogelsang (2020). He says: "Identity then becomes a balancing of different identity parts in different networks." (Vogelsang 2020, p. 200).

15.3 The Compilation of Groups: The Application of the Typology of Analytical Psychology

The continued popularity of the MBTI (Myers-Briggs-Type Indicator) (cf. Myers 1985) in personnel selection in business is amusing: How can it be that a personality psychology based on the typology of C. G. Jung is applied in the sober world of business? Both Jung and Freud were predominantly opposed to the idea of groups, suspecting primarily an increase in regressive processes. Trigant Burrow, an analysand of Jung, is the namesake of group analysis (cf. Alder 2016). He influenced the thinking of Bion and Foulkes. He was interested in the "own socially conditioned identity" as an obstacle and opportunity. A topic for Jung and Freud was also the fear of the power of group leadership: For the initial phase of groups, it is necessary to deal with this. The threat to individual narcissism is often responded to with group narcissism ("We are a special, unique group"). The leaders should also beware of such hypertrophy.

Vitality in Groups through Proper Compilation

The typology within Jung's Analytical Psychology has identified a category system with the poles of introversion and extraversion as well as the dimensions of thinking, feeling, sensing, and intuiting as significant sizes of human functional styles. There are manifold mixed forms. When assembling a group, it makes sense to have as many manifestations of these dimensions as possible. Since the group members complement each other (also unconsciously), it is beneficial for identification processes if both similarity and difference are represented. The longing for connection is satisfied when the generally known "Noah's Ark principle" is applied in the compilation of a group: Always two participants of a "kind" should be able to connect and ally with each other, this reduces the level of fear. This can involve the classic manifestations of old character and personality psychology such as anxious, obsessive, depressive or hysterical (today histrionic) or even narcissistic personality structures—or the aforementioned typological features. Following Jungian terminology and recommendation, in a typical therapeutic group of eight participants, at least two pronounced thinking types, two people with a dominant feeling function, two sensing people and two primarily intuitively functioning participants would be gathered, each with one extraverted and one introverted emphasis. This ideal-typical and never fully realizable compilation often makes a group process easier, smoother, and more lively, as the differences naturally mark boundaries and invite discussion from different perspectives.

References

Alder, S (2016) Die Geschichte der Gruppenanalyse in der Analytischen Psychologie von 1957 bis zur Gegenwart. In: Schimkus, M; Stuck, U (2016) Selbst, Ich und Wir. Brandes & Apsel Verlag, Frankfurt/M

Braun, C (2003) Individuation und Gruppenpsychotherapie—ein Widerspruch in sich? Jahrbuch f. Gruppenanalyse 9: 138–160

Dalal, F (1998) Taking the Group Seriously. Jessica Kingsley Publishers, London
Dorst, B (2016) Der Archetyp der Gruppe. In: Schimkus, M; Stuck, U (2016) Selbst, Ich und Wir. Brandes & Apsel Verlag, Frankfurt/M
Illouz E (2009) Die Errettung der modernen Seele. Suhrkamp, Frankfurt/M
Jung, C G (1995) Praxis der Psychotherapie. In: GW 8. Patmos, Düsseldorf
Lesmeister, R (2009) Selbst und Individuation. Brandes & Apsel Verlag, Frankfurt/M
Münch, V (2021) Die therapeutische Haltung. Kohlhammer, Stuttgart
Myers, I B; McCauley, M H (1985) Manual: A guide to the development and use of the Myers-Briggs-Type-Indicator. Consulting Psychologists Press, Palo Alto
Otscheret, L (2005) Dialektik ohne Dialog. In: Otscheret, L, Braun, C (2005) Im Dialog mit dem Anderen. Brandes & Apsel Verlag, Frankfurt/M
Stuck, U (2016) Plädoyer für den Gruppengedanken in der Analytischen Psychologie. In: Schimkus, M; Stuck, U (2016) Selbst, Ich und Wir. Brandes & Apsel Verlag, Frankfurt/M
Vogelsang, F (2020) Soziale Verbundenheit. Verlag Karl Alber, Freiburg/München
Yalom, I D (2016) Theorie und Praxis der Gruppenpsychotherapie. Klett-Cotta, Stuttgart
Yalom, I D (2005) Die Schopenhauer-Kur. btb, München

Large Groups

16

Abstract

The dynamics in small groups can be better understood when compared to the dynamics of large groups. Here, similarities as well as differences can be found. Above all, the different levels of fear are crucial. The affiliation of individuals to different societal and personal large and small groups creates a complex interplay and also a field of tension, which must be understood at least to some extent if one wants to understand the reactions of individuals to their fellow human beings. This also applies to (analytical) psychotherapy in groups.

Large groups are, depending on interpretation, groups of over 15 participants and not yet mass movements. They are usually defined by a framework such as a club or an institution, like a company, and by common underlying goals and tasks. However, large groups are particularly susceptible to tensions, which usually arise from the fears that build up faster in them than in small groups. The fact that more fears circulate in large groups simply results from the fact that it becomes impossible in them to know everyone, at least everyone approximately equally well. The other as the unknown mobilizes fears in us of attacks on our identity, our worldview, our feelings. Since direct personal contact in the large group becomes more difficult, conflicts can potentially be negotiated less well and there is a latently high vulnerability of the individual group member.

Institutionalized Large Groups

The typical large group in the experience horizon of psychotherapists is the planned, guided large group within the framework of conferences or gatherings of professional societies, training institutes or other associations of the professional group. The instrument of the guided large group has been successfully used for decades for "psychohygiene" and organizational development at

V. Münch, *Group Experience as a Resource*,
https://doi.org/10.1007/978-3-662-70864-4_16

psychotherapeutic training institutes, in professional and trade associations, and in regional, even international formats. Examples would be the Nazareth conferences in Israel and various follow-up formats with British, Israeli, Palestinian and German participants or the large groups initiated within the framework of the Ukrainian-Russian-German trialog conferences, which continue in online format even in times of war. This event was initiated by Stephan Alder, a meritorious Jungian colleague. In this context, conflicts, fears and hitherto unprocessed issues, often also historically relevant and affecting all present, are brought to light and can thus be better perceived and integrated by all.

The typical large group in the contexts mentioned above then comprises about 35–150 participants. People sit in a sufficiently large room either in concentric circles or in a seating arrangement arranged in a spiral. Therefore, the acoustics can sometimes become a problem, which then forces individual "soft speakers" to have to present their concerns louder and more clearly. In clinical contexts, there are the most diverse groups and group sizes, which sometimes leads to confusion, as the different processes in small and large groups and the conflicts arising from them receive too little attention. Groups of over 15 participants are subject to a different dynamic: due to the individual's overload to be able to establish any kind of contact with the others. This activates more primitive defense mechanisms to cope with one's own insecurity. Working in and with large groups is, according to Wilke (2017), a rewarding task despite all obstacles: The underlying conflicts, resentments and neurotic fixations and identifications visible there hinder the progress and effective work of institutions of all kinds. Unprocessed content leads to the various subgroups producing splitting and projection phenomena, which can ultimately lead to the collapse of the institution itself. Nitsun (2014) has shown that the integration of destructive tendencies in the group context is highly significant in order to find a lasting productive exchange with each other. This may seem paradoxical, but it corresponds to the tension of opposites in the psyche, as described by Jung (see Jung 1995).

Change through the Regressive State

The significantly higher level of fear in large groups leads to a stronger tendency to regress, activating more primitive defense mechanisms. However, this allows the group events to influence much deeper, more elemental levels of the psychic structure. Here, the dynamics and mode of action, which are also effective in small groups, albeit in a weakened form, are demonstrated using the example of large group dynamics. Regressed to an earlier functional level, the interventions of the leaders and the group are all the more effective as they encounter a more open, vulnerable individual, here embedded in a regressed, vulnerable group. Just how much the development of groups and in groups depends on this mutual deep interweaving becomes clear. The fear of the group is the fear of the individual and both entities, if we tentatively consider them separately, influence the well-being of the respective other side. It behaves in large groups then analogously as in small groups: The joint enduring, witnessing and articulating of difficult affective contents leads to a strengthening of the ego, a greater tolerance of frustration and a decrease in inner tension, as fewer frightening contents of one's own as well as common unconscious have to be repressed. Under certain circumstances, however, a more active approach will be required from the conductors.

In large groups, conflicts also come to light that have a large group-specific, indeed mass psychological character. Thus, contemporary historical and historical developments of a societal, economic and political nature also have an impact on the topics addressed. Behind current conflicts of individual members, who identificatorily bring the inner conflict of the group "to performance" as protagonists, there are usually also difficult historical events, war experiences, losses, the shadow aspects of one's own organization.

Various Settings of Group Application

In group-analytical training as well as in some intensive therapeutic formats, several small groups and a large group with the members of all other small groups take place on one day. The different dynamics in small and large groups are very revealing and tell something about the way in which the same people react differently in different group contexts and what defense is used. This has an integrative aspect, as it becomes more conscious to both the other participants and the persons concerned themselves, what influences groups and their compositions can have on their experience and behavior. If conflicts in a small group cannot be well maintained, they "spill over" into the large group, which contains both opportunities and risks. The risk lies in a stronger polarization due to the mentioned higher level of fear, the opportunity lies in the possibility of coalition formation, the mutual balancing through complementary aspects, which, verbalized by the participants, are able to illuminate a fact more precisely.

Example

A good example of the meaningfulness of external supervision in clinical contexts are the different interests and backgrounds of nursing staff and psychologists and doctors. While there is usually a rather homogeneous opinion in team meetings and within individual professional groups, there is often a mixed mood regarding the opinion about the others. In joint large groups, these conflicts, which are often based on (projected) fears and prejudices, ignorance and lack of exchange, can be mitigated. ◂

In institutionally anchored large groups, such as the entirety of those employed in a clinic, the situation is determined both by the factual structural conditions and the personal psychodynamics. Often there are power-political or financial dependencies that are the cause of dissatisfaction, anger and overload. Narcissistic pathologies of leadership figures are often suspected behind closed doors, so creative solutions and compromises, often in the sense of an internal change of attitude or perspective of those affected, are in demand. In this context, narcissistic leadership personalities are characterized by their often pronounced ambition and their almost complete inability to deal socially appropriately with group phenomena (cf. Externbrinck and Keil 2017).

Organizational Development in the Field of Tension

If large groups, which include all those affected, are installed in these contexts, there is often more resistance than expected, as it is suspected that this group experience is offered with a controlling-manipulative intention to achieve the corporate goal or to rehabilitate the finances. Especially in professional fields like clinics, for which many clinical experts rather suggest the principle of "care for existence" than a monetary, profit-oriented orientation, it is particularly difficult to establish open-ended groups. If the boss is present, the cards are initially bad that there will be sustainable changes, as the inner fears are activated most strongly. The management can then bring forward as an alibi that they have offered formats to "get into conversation with each other".

Profit Maximization in Healthcare

In psychotherapeutic-psychosomatic clinical contexts, where the system also aims at profit maximization, employees sometimes feel like agents of goals that do not converge with their own, often humanistically oriented values. Their expertise is often not appreciated enough, the performance of the psychotherapists is not seen and compensated appropriately. In this respect, there is often an unspoken contradiction between the goals of therapeutic interventions and the goals of the institution. The uncertainty under which the employees suffer ultimately becomes noticeable in their work: patients notice this and can cause considerable confusion with their defense mechanisms and contribute to even more disillusionment. One could also interpret it this way: With their "non-recovery", the patients give a fitting comment to a dysfunctional system. Namely, by experiencing the treating persons in a group in which they do not really feel self-empowered and thus can serve little as a role model. There are numerous examples of how burdensome institutional tensions in facilities and clinics can affect the well-being and dynamics among patients and between treating persons and patients.

Example

In an outpatient addiction therapy facility, the therapists always perceived the management's profit motive as paramount. Patients were summoned and admitted, even when the capacities for this were actually no longer available. This made the individuals concerned feel helpless and angry. External supervision was able to help bring some issues to light and thus make them more bearable. In another outpatient facility, the management initially did not introduce clear rules for violations of treatment contracts, leading to numerous transgressions and various disagreements about the correct sanctions. The background was also a profit-oriented, too rapid growth of a still young facility. This led to high staff turnover, which seriously threatened the stability of the team for a long time. External supervision gradually led to a calming down, as the team and its leader could strengthen themselves and increasingly make their presence felt to the management. ◄

16.1 Groups and Ideology

Example

During the Covid-19 pandemic, some members of my analytical groups also showed severe stress symptoms in the face of the many restrictions on daily life imposed by the authorities. Furthermore, there were also people who did not want to join the general vaccination call. The reactions among my patients ranged from vehement rejection and identification with conspiracy ideologies like Q-Anon to well-argued rejection of vaccination as such. Many others seemed rather fearful and compliant. Concern was expressed primarily in view of the fears in society, which were repeatedly experienced as strongly fueled. There was a great desire for reassurance and confidence. ◄

The pandemic vividly demonstrated how societal large group processes affect the therapeutic small group. However, this happens *always* en passant, without being greatly noticed or thematized. Here, however, this connection came to light as if under a magnifying glass. Ideologies in the sense of sociologist Norbert Elias (1997) serve a society as a "meaning-giving glue". Belief in one or the other "truth" helps to reduce fears. Fears of chaos, overwhelm, and unstructuredness, which every group has to deal with, are thus regulated (cf. Dalal 1998). From a psychodynamic perspective, however, chaos threatens more from the direction of the (own) unconscious. But the unconscious, if it appears sufficiently unpleasant, is gladly projected and perceived as coming from outside, such as the fear that society could descend into anarchy.

Psychological and Antipsychological Ideologemes

It seems important that everyone should assume that we have identifications with ideologies. Psychoanalysts should have such at least with the basic assumptions of psychoanalysis. However, this means that the conversations and discussions in therapeutic groups also follow an ideology, which of course as a "therapeutic ideology" is also questionable here and there. Illouz (2009) has dealt extensively with this topic from a sociological perspective and described the disadvantages of a psychologization of society. What she means by this and what I believe should be reflected upon is the fact that too much therapeutic thinking and psychological vocabulary can also creep into a therapeutic group. This often happens in the service of an intellectualizing defense. The often diverse therapeutic experiences of the patients and the reading of psychological advice books influence perception, experience, and language. This can lead to participants in groups initially arguing on the basis of such catchphrase-like and schematic ways of thinking. Advice to other group participants in that case is also popular. Only gradually does it become clear in group processes that empathy and listening can achieve more than many a hasty piece of advice. Because what applies to oneself does not necessarily have to be valid for others. Here, respect for difference, despite all the similarity of conflict themes, becomes increasingly greater in the course of the group. The fact that as a therapist one sometimes also gets competition in terms of psychological expertise is another matter. It can also facilitate the work in the group if thinking and interaction already take a certain therapeutic direction, without having to constantly remind this as a conductor. However, there is always a need for differentiation. On another note, the generally often antipsychological attitude of the performance society, which is not interested in uncovering repressed material, is a concern. These tendencies can be counteracted in therapeutic groups by establishing awareness and reciprocity of contacts.

The Farewell from the Group

The departure of individuals from a therapy group confronts everyone in the group with their ego ideal. One must face the limitations of what has been achieved and the finiteness of all relationships. This also puts pressure on the therapeutic ideal, which assumes a completeness of the achievement of treatment goals. As a result, achieved progress is somewhat relativized and related to other areas of life that may be harder to change. Essentially, it always comes down to finding a balance between the gain in creative power and the acceptance of the inevitable. In contrast, interventions by not very therapy-experienced group members sometimes have a somewhat apodictic character. Only over the course of a group, also along the experienced farewells without resolution of all conflicts of the concerned, a greater tolerance of ambiguity towards the "facts of life" develops (cf. Money-Kyrle 1971), especially towards finiteness.

Example

In one of my long-term groups, after a holiday-related absence and break, a discussion arose about what the group "brings". It became clear that beyond all individual progress, limits become visible. Not least, it was discussed that everyone has to contribute in order to receive something. Without overcoming shame and fears of showing oneself and becoming vulnerable, the others cannot show empathy either. Because they cannot know what *exactly* the situations and conditions are that burden or trigger the other participants. Initially admitting that there are topics that have not yet been addressed was a first step towards greater openness. ◄

16.2 Therapists Learn in Groups

Firstly, it is pleasing that group self-experience is found again as a mandatory component in the new psychotherapist training in Germany. It is a pity that this is partly at the expense of individual self-experience or teaching therapy or teaching analysis, but it is a signal. In addition, the freedom to apply and better payment for group therapies have led to a significant increase in group therapies carried out in statutory care within a short time. Supervisions in groups and case study seminars also play a larger role in training and further education. Here, therapists in training learn from the model, can exchange ideas about characteristic problems in the early stages of the therapeutic career and thus relieve themselves. This should also lead to the therapists in private practice networking in their later professional everyday life and regularly taking intervision with and supervision from colleagues, i.e. in groups. This is usually the case. However, for such an intervision group to be able to unfold its helpful potential, a positive group experience is necessary. The openness and transparency that are necessary to report on the difficulties in treating certain patients—the inevitable personal involvement and the realization of one's own vulnerability and mistakes—all this requires a trusting framework and a great deal of emotional security. There should be no fear of evaluation and criticism, rather one should be able to rely on the goodwill and understanding of colleagues.

16.3 Societal Divisions and a Remedy

In the SRF podcast "Sternstunde Philosophie", sociologist Oliver Nachtwey (2023) refers to the phenomenon of "lateral thinkers" and attributes to them an unprocessed injury as a result of a misunderstood concept of individual freedom. Those who have had good family experiences are aware that their own freedom ends at the boundary of others' freedom. This could be well observed during the coronavirus pandemic. His paradoxically seeming thesis "Freedom can primarily be experienced together" (Nachtwey, 2023), finds its justification in the statement: "Individual freedom always occurs in conjunction with the freedom of other people." In the book *Injured Freedom*, Nachtwey, together with his colleague and partner Carolin Amlinger, elaborates that we are always already group beings, even before we are aware of it. Groups first enable individual freedoms by opening up spaces for encounters and creative creations. The freedom of the individual and the functioning of society are, in a certain way, antagonists, but only at first glance.

New Group Formats for the Divided Society

In this sense, Stuck (2016) also argues when he writes: "The group therapeutic field [is] an experiential space that gives the individual group member the opportunity to examine the offered thought concepts and thought spaces for their credibility, consistency, and reliability. … The group therapeutic approach … stands … for a democratic, respecting the other as different, impetus." (ibid., p. 76). With group therapy, there is a laboratory where one can study in detail how individuality (the never completed "end product" of a development), individuation (the process of this development), and group identity are intertwined. If you look closer, it is always other people who enable my experience of freedom. Even the author of this book, who is sitting here alone with his laptop, is not alone. He writes for an (hopefully existing) imaginary audience, he writes because there is a publisher behind him who has agreed to publish his ideas. And he writes from the resource of his own positive and also negative group experiences.

Adrienne Weiß and Mandy Koplin and other colleagues have set up something in Munich that is currently happening in many cities around the world: As psychoanalysts, they provide open groups (e.g., "city group" in Munich) in which citizens of various origins and with different views can engage in exchange. Here, forums are to be created that can counteract the tendency towards societal division. At the same time, the analytical way of thinking and competence are made known and used in a popularized form. The idea behind it: Especially analytical competence with its tolerance of ambiguity, with its ability to listen, not to judge, to promote development, seems to be what society currently needs.

References

Dalal, F (1998) Taking the Group Seriously. Jessica Kingsley Publishers, London

Elias, N (1997) Über den Prozess der Zivilisation. Suhrkamp, Frankfurt/M

Externbrink, K, Keil, M (2017) Narzissmus, Machiavellismus und Psychopathie in Organisationen. Theorien, Methoden und Befunde zur dunklen Triade. Springer, Heidelberg

Illouz E (2009) Die Errettung der modernen Seele. Suhrkamp, Frankfurt/M

Jung, C G (1995) Gesammelte Werke, VIII. Patmos, Düsseldorf

Money-Kyrle, R (1971) The aim of psychoanalysis. International Journal of Psychoanalysis 52: 103–106

Nachtwey, O (2022) Selbstbestimmung vs. staatliche Bevormundung.| Sternstunde Philosophie. SRF Kultur: https://www.youtube.com/watch?app=desktop&v=Ye3Y2Mzi7Lo Stand: 26.09.2023

Nitsun, M (2014) The Anti-Group. Routledge, London

Stuck, U (2016) Plädoyer für den Gruppengedanken in der Analytischen Psychologie. In Schimkus, M Stuck U (2016) Selbst, Ich und Wir. Brandes & Apsel, Frankfurt

Wilke, G (2017) Ordnung und Chaos in Gruppen. Lit-Verlag, Wien, Zürich

Society in the Group 17

Abstract

Genetic, biographical, and societal influences converge in the individual and find a unique psychological expression. Historical processes, migration movements, and ideological mass movements have a significant impact on the structuring and well-being of individuals. Analytical group psychotherapy should consider these factors if it wants to arrive at a realistic assessment of the situation of patients and if it is looking for ways to strengthen the influence of individuals on their inner experiences and external behavior.

The past years have brought about significant changes and new insights for group therapists and their patients. The much larger extent to which societal phenomena have penetrated individual consciousness can almost be described as traumatic. At the very least, people's attention is shifting. It always involves the perception that our previous life in our Western societies appears to be sensitively disturbed (in a double sense) or seems to be coming to an end. The effects of the Covid-19 pandemic were most evident in group work. Groups were not allowed to meet for months if the minimum distances between participants could not be maintained. Wearing masks made communication more difficult, both in terms of facial perception and in articulation and acoustic understanding of what was being said. Towards the end of the pandemic, other societal discourses became more present in many groups. Thus, group participants repeatedly raised the issue of climate change. Optimism and confidence in the future seemed to have at least clouded over, helplessness and depression were spreading. On the one hand, this questions the purpose of group therapy, because what sense would it make to recover only to continue in a "sick" and unsolidary society that has no future? On the other hand, the lack of solidarity in society could indeed be compensated for in the groups.

V. Münch, *Group Experience as a Resource*,
https://doi.org/10.1007/978-3-662-70864-4_17

Many participants were very grateful for the group, as they had few other group experiences during the pandemic.

The Normality of Societal Topics in Groups

Towards the end of the pandemic, not only was the climate crisis frequently addressed directly or indirectly as a burdensome apocalyptic vision, but also the war in Ukraine. The diverse images of destruction, real, currently occurring and possible future destruction can be shared in groups and made somewhat more bearable. However, the question arises to what extent the neutrality of the analytical situation and the focus on the dynamics of the individuals and especially the group is not abandoned with such a broadening of perspective. It will not be surprising if I argue at this point to sensibly include these influences, to give them space and to jointly investigate their influence on mental life (cf. Hirblinger 2023). Especially in groups, it would sometimes be grotesque if the world were excluded in this way, if conflicts and narratives that unfold in the group were thus again repressed. Systemically viewed, these are often enough expressions of scenarios that, mediated by real experiences in and with society and the great influence of social media, co-determine our daily consciousness.

Example

A patient who had been in the group for a long time considered his own troubles and issues to be less relevant than those of others, thus justifying his reticence. Only gradually did his dissatisfaction with his situation become clear. On the one hand, his abstinence reflected his usual behavior in social situations, on the other hand, he also brought up the issue of his future fears in the face of the "world", also against the background of his situation as a father of two children. Here it became apparent how general fears and helplessness overlapped with a midlife crisis. The patient lacked the biographical experience of a supportive and crisis-resilient father. The general crisis and the internal pressure it triggered were for him a reason to take his own crisis more seriously and to verbalize it. ◄

In addition, there is another important observation regarding the world outside the door of group psychotherapy: Many of the participants in (group) therapies are confronted with news and reports from the internet that interest, occupy and fascinate them, but also captivate, frighten, unsettle or anger them, right up until the group sessions. But how can confidence now arise within the group framework when news seems to be tumbling over each other in their pessimistic worldview, which makes one believe that nothing in the world is permanent or gives cause for hope? After all, internal, biographically caused restlessness and fears are also constantly reactivated by these constant external triggers. So, should there be the advice "no drinking, no internet" after the group sessions?

In the podcast "Lanz and Precht" (2023) with journalist Markus Lanz and philosopher Richard David Precht from 27.01.2023, the two discuss whether the media (also concerning my patients) spreading alarmism and pessimism is not too one-sided. Lanz quotes the Swedish doctor Hans Rosling (2023), who can show that many parameters, such as poverty and hunger in the world, are factually in retreat. Looking neutrally at the conflict thus presented, one wonders whether both developments are not running in parallel. Then it would even be the case, in a perverse way, that some objectively demonstrable improvement only appears to us as such. Because the consequences of increasing prosperity do have an impact on possessions, quality of life and even lifespan in the "global north". At the same time, however, the increasing consumption promotes a negative climate balance and this in turn increased destruction of nature. In the end, with increasing knowledge about the complex interaction of ecosystems, we are more and more in a consciousness of fragility, guilt, at least responsibility for a way of life whose shadow aspects we have long kept hidden from ourselves. This burdens people quite individually, especially when they are prone to feelings of guilt and quick assumption of responsibility for the mistakes of others.

Intergenerationality

The surrounding society thus finds its way into group events on various levels. On the one hand, there are societal upheavals and crises that reach individuals through the media. They question lifestyles and life plans, as well as fantasies about one's own position in society, what can be achieved or desired in life. All these aspects are put to the test and questioned in groups. Therefore, they practically affect the emotional and psychological positioning within therapeutic processes. Accepting one's own psychological and physical life also involves finding one's own position and role in intergenerational and thus societal exchange.

Example

Once when the older members of the group were absent, the middle-aged participants of one of my groups engaged in a discussion about different individual and generational differences in the perception of accelerated technical and societal development. There was a lot of understanding for the older people's alienation, which also showed that the relative "loneliness" of one's own position in the succession of generations and the decidedly different experience and opinion could be tolerated. The more advanced detachment from parental images in some, and the still faltering detachment in others, was vividly reflected in the statements. Among those with more therapy experience, there was more serenity, humor, and self-acceptance, but also the ability to name remaining conflicts and fears. ◄

17.1 Social Origin and Group

An important thought, which Dalal (1998) also repeatedly addresses, concerns the reflection of societal conditions in the psychological structure of individuals. He does not want to consider these individuals separately from these influences.

In his view, expectations, desires, needs, and their possibilities of satisfaction are encoded and passed on in the social unconscious. At this point, however, class-specific experiences also emerge, pointing to differences in mental processing possibilities in different societal milieus. Mental illness, which is generally attributed to parental influence in the analytical milieu, by definition takes place in a basic family situation that is embedded in education and working conditions to which the parents were and are exposed. These, in turn, are embedded in societal conditions that concern educational justice, occupational safety, and discourses about the influence of the working environment (groups!) on people. The distress of the parents often goes back to the distress of the grandparents, who were war children or participants and could usually process their traumas only very rudimentarily. The legacy of history and thus the reality of societal large groups permeates the psyche of the individual and should not be thought of separately from it. Developing an awareness of this in groups promotes a sense of one's own place in history, one's own responsibility, but also an awareness of the cause of one's own limitations. As the group participants get to know the stories of the others better over time and also their own story and the reactions of the others to it, they notice these differences. At the same time, paradoxically, what connects everyone beyond the differences is also noticed. The act of reciprocity in listening and speaking establishes this homogenization and alignment. A new group feeling emerges beyond the brought along, often unconscious identifications with social classes, groups, and origins.

Example

Especially when new group participants are members of social professions such as doctors or therapists, it can temporarily happen that the other group participants address them in their expertise. This situation can particularly occur when trainees in psychotherapy carry out their group sessions in a mixed, existing group with "normal" patients. However, it is usually the case that a grown group has a good sense for the fact that the others want to be seen as people and not in their function. If newcomers hide behind their profession and give advice from their professional competence, the conductors will of course also pick up this rivaling and defensive movement in some way, should the group not have already done so. ◂

The often subtle, yet clear differences in dealing with conflicts, feelings, and general human concerns that exist among members of different social milieus are subliminally present in a therapeutic group as well. The "verbalization of emotional experience content", a characteristic of humanistic conversation therapy often found in the middle class, is unfamiliar to some from less well-off social backgrounds. Here, perhaps the rule is that one does not "air one's dirty laundry", that one presents oneself as non-committal and tough. Conversely, those who have perhaps already excessively engaged in self-exploration and self-expression, so that it sometimes already takes on a defensive character again, can benefit from the direct, perhaps initially coarser-seeming affect communication of “simpler” participants. Since it can once be about achieving more access to affects and more communication of the same, another time about better perceiving one’s own affects but also controlling them more appropriately, a group can serve to complement these different ways of dealing with affects and their communication identificatorily.

17.2 Cultural Complexes

One way to articulate what shapes and determines large group processes and societies is the concept of “Cultural Complexes”. Jörg Rasche (2016) has popularized and worked on this concept by the American Tom Singer in the German-speaking world. Since the 1980s, psychotherapists from the Jungian “camp” have also been concerned about the ecological consequences of our economic activities and the dangers posed by technology to nature and wildlife. Springer writes that in the face of the then rampant fear of annihilation by nuclear war (which was recently updated), “a group is not simply practical and meaningful support of one’s own actions, but it is *fundamentally* necessary” (cf. Springer 1988, p. 31). In a group, one’s own “encounter with destructiveness” is possible through the assumption of different positions. Therefore, Springer also asserts that group self-experience is an appropriate access for the part of the population suffering from severe personality disorders. This is even more true if one wants to attribute these diagnoses to society itself. These thoughts make clear the high potential that groups can be attributed within societies and how dangerous it can be to underestimate this influence. Since psychoanalytic thinking always aims to understand how the existential fear inherent in humans (ultimately of one’s own finiteness) can be minimized and sometimes better defended, the apparent security of ideologies, as they help to solidify group identities in the current identity discourse, seems worth investigating.

Belief and Religion
Religious and spiritual belief systems move us in the deepest and most lasting way. These are shared by many people in their own unique way. The rituals of a religion provide a large number of people with security and a framework to give our existence on this earth a meaning, an interpretation. Even the atheist sets such a rule by “believing” in the non-existence of a god. Maintaining hope and faith in the future and formulating visions for a better future seems more urgent than ever. The concern of my colleague Jörg Rasche, which he expresses in his latest book *Menetekel* (2022), is justified, but it is becoming increasingly difficult for the older among us to believe in the power of change that is nourished by faith in the future. The younger among us, who have this future ahead of them, develop surprisingly positive perspectives that also influence their daily lives. Networking in a completely new way, namely on a much larger scale, is the everyday life of the younger generation. Here, digitization offers potential for synergies that may overshadow all progress made so far. Groups in which young people interested

in common goals meet, carry risks of one-sidedness and secession, but also the potential for the development of new ideas for living together and sustainable development of humans and nature. How groups can be understood as a social size and continuity, as a force against the overwhelming societal change, is described by Geyer (2023). He attributes to the "therapeutic group not only the character of a normative institution … but it could also be called political" (Geyer 2023, p. 11). For him, the work of a group moves between the neuroticizing social context of the patients and the conflicts in democratic societies. It is about not taking sides and not identifying too quickly with divisive phenomena such as one-sided world-views. However, this could also include the theoretical, psychological assumptions (such as a too narrowly defined concept of the "individual") that sometimes make therapists themselves blind to operations. The ethical questions that go along with this could then be discussed more intensively in groups of experts.

References

Dalal, F (1998) Taking the Group Seriously. Jessica Kingsley Publishers, London

Geyer, M (2023) Die Gruppe als normative Instanz im Wandel der Zeiten. Gruppenpsychother. Gruppendynamik 59: 1, 2–16

Hirblinger, A (2023) Über Tabus im psychoanalytischen Dialog und das Gebot des Einbezugs gesellschaftlicher Realitäten als Quelle psychischen Leidens. In: Ztsch Forum für Psychoanalyse, Heft 3/2023, Springer, Heidelberg

Lanz und Precht (Ausgabe 73) https://open.spotify.com/episode/2CbCnVVhcLJlMs4B0y73Rv) Stand: 27.01.2023

Rasche, J, Singer, T (2016) Europe's Many Souls: Exploring Cultural Complexes and Identities. Spring Journal Books, New Orleans

Rasche, J (2022) Menetekel. Königshausen und Neumann, Würzburg

Rosling, H (2023) Factfulness—wie wir lernen, die Welt so zu sehen, wie sie wirklich ist. Ullstein, Berlin

Springer, A (1988) In: Dieckmann, H, Springer A (Eds) Weltzerstörung—Selbstzerstörung. Walter, Düsseldorf

18 Limits of the Effectiveness of Group Therapies

Abstract

Group therapies, of course, cannot override or even make understandable every dynamic. There are individuals and situations where one should terminate participation in a group or the group itself to prevent further harm. The humility in the face of one's own fallibility and one's own "not knowing" of those involved in group therapy (in the sense of Bion) is essential. It can be helpful to remind oneself of this in stressful and conflict situations in groups in order to gain distance. The acceptance of boundaries also always points to what is still possible on this side of the boundary or has not turned for the worse.

Groups have their disadvantages, especially when they are inadequately managed and moderated. The framework of a group is crucial for its success. The fundamental mistrust that groups are met with from the narcissistic side must be repeatedly addressed and empathetically addressed. Otherwise, too large parts of the personality remain in their isolation and resentment, and the person concerned remains below the possibilities of life design. Combination therapy (see Sect. 10.5) offers many possibilities in this regard, as it can be experienced how differently situations are experienced in the dyad on the one hand and the triadic constellations of the group on the other hand. I personally know several people, both as patients and in my circle of friends, who in my opinion have not benefited much from a too one-sided therapy. This applies to both the idealization of individual treatment and group treatment. Often I would have wished both experiences for the person concerned. The internal comparison between the dyadic experience of the individual setting and the triadic, multiple of the group context is as stimulating and development-promoting as the oscillation between the psychic positions "paranoid-schizoid" and "depressive" described by Melanie Klein's successors.

V. Münch, *Group Experience as a Resource*,
https://doi.org/10.1007/978-3-662-70864-4_18

In my opinion, no setting can assume that it can unfold the sole power of interpretation or integration effect. There are always constellations that may require a combination of both settings. This should also be the subject of further research dedicated to the effectiveness of combination therapy. In addition, it applies: Group psychotherapies have different effects on every patient. Everyone starts from a different starting point of their psychic position. As we have seen, it is not only essential to realize that destructive forces are always at work in all group processes. These must be recognized, endured, and overcome in their own way in order to be able to carry out further constructive work in groups. Sometimes, however, it is also necessary to question and then dissolve outdated group structures or a problematic integration of groups into certain organizations and institutions in order to find new, more functional group forms. A widespread example causing much suffering are the institutional dysfunctions of the large group Church, which have favored abuse of power and resulting maldevelopments.

The Group and Society as Triangulation Aid

The same applies to economic actors: The relentless pressure of a critical public towards fossil energy companies is obviously necessary to bring about only small changes. The billion-dollar campaigns of the oil multinationals, on the other hand, have at least managed to convey to the individual the concept of the "personal CO_2 footprint", also to disguise the collective and structural exercise of power. In addition to the challenge posed by destructive group forces, whether in the context of group psychotherapy or in connection with the global institutional players of the energy industry, there are hidden dynamics within the individual, usually reinforced in the life history, that let us know that they will not simply disappear through interventions, nor through waiting. The opposite is the case. Even in the favorable case of successful psychotherapeutic treatment, which may have set many changes in motion in the inner and outer life of those treated: often there remain residual areas of crisis-like escalations, of "trigger situations", which can sometimes be difficult for the persons concerned to master. As shown in the examples above, masochistic and narcissistic processing in conflict situations or in difficult to bear situations of shame and disappointment continue to prevail. The group remains a lifelong challenge for these people. Despite a great longing for belonging and participation, the fear of losing the objects and at the same time the never really achieved individuality remains in these contexts and wants to be endured and mourned.

Dealing with Groups as a Lifelong Theme

For these people, the difficulties in internal triangulation pose a perpetual challenge. The retreat to narcissistic ways of experiencing is put to the test every time a group situation arises. In other words: What has served the narcissistically deficient person as compensation for humiliation, shame, and failure over long periods of life, namely ideas of their own invulnerability, grandiosity, and uniqueness, is relativized and questioned in the face of encounters and confrontations in a group. What brings joy to other people, namely sharing this joy with other people, is precisely what poses a danger to the narcissistically constituted person. The fact that it should be so much easier to derive satisfaction from contact with other people, but also from oneself, hurts these people precisely at the moment when they could let the new experience approach them. The whole complexity of one's own thought and experience world turns out to be superfluous when it comes to the simple things of human life. Fittingly, narcissistic people tend to retreat into professions distant from people, into interests where they create abstract worlds of thought. In the past, these were perhaps more often the philosophical faculties, today perhaps more often the sector of programming, coding, AI (cf. Ullman, 1997, 2018).

The Contrast between Narcissism and Group Experience
One could also say that it is so difficult to truly feel that one is supported by a community, that one can rely on others, that one does not have to organize and control everything oneself in order to lead a satisfied and average life. As already mentioned in the section on narcissistic patients in groups (see Sect. 11.1), narcissists experience groups more as a threat than as an enrichment of their identity. They cannot feel that they are simultaneously both part of a group and an individual. Their consciousness always slips too quickly from one pole to the other. They fear disappearing in a group, which can mobilize terrible and elemental psychic fears of annihilation (which usually originate from early childhood). Therefore, they avoid and deny any dependence or need in relation to others. They often withdraw from social contacts and pursue their thoughts and plans. When they come into contact with other people, if it is unavoidable, they tend to want to control them.

Thus, one can also observe that a mentally functioning person always manages to achieve the acceptance of the group surrounding him. Precisely what seems self-evident to us, namely integration into the social environment, must appear to narcissistic patients in general, but especially in the challenging context of group psychotherapy, as an impossibility. This is most evident at the beginning of treatments, when the prospect of group participation is psychologically feared, as one cannot imagine benefiting from contact with others. In contrast, images and ideas of psychological abuse, boredom, the inferiority of others, their "babble" dominate. A well-known defensive maneuver to cope with these fears is the projection of one's own discarded, shameful, aggressive parts onto the others in a group. Perhaps this exaggerated defense is also familiar to us from everyday circumstances: When one enters a new, unknown group of people, the feeling of insecurity is the rule. For a short time, as long as no real contact is established, one can sometimes hear people gossiping about the impossible others, their clothing, their behavior, their presence. Often these negative projections disappear very quickly as soon as a first contact has taken place and one finds, surprisingly to oneself, that these "others", who were just devalued for one's own self-stabilization, are actually quite nice.

18.1 Group is Not Equal to Group

Example

How differently groups can be perceived and how much this also seems to depend on the behavior of their leadership personalities was once illustrated to me by a patient who attended a ward group and a theme-centered group during a clinic treatment that interrupted continuous group therapy. The clinic setting made this group participation mandatory. The patient experienced the interventions of the younger therapists as intrusive and insensitive. She was repeatedly asked to report on her traumatic childhood, although she had justifiably refused. The patient's understandable resistance to self-disclosure in a relatively unfamiliar environment was obviously not taken very seriously, but was confronted head-on. ◂

So for therapists who offer and conduct groups, it is about bridging the following dilemma: On the one hand, they know that groups can be perceived as frightening, and they also know about the destructive forces that can be inherent in groups. Many patients have experienced this in their childhood. Their experiences range from dysfunctional families and experiences of bullying to overwhelming contexts in the learning area. On the other hand, as an experienced group therapist, I also know about the connecting, social and human power that can be released in every group. The belief in these healing powers, which only become alive in the exchange between people, is in my opinion essential for group processes to succeed and for people to be able to take positive experiences from groups. Therapists can also rejoice in the unfolding of these powers and thus participate in these developments. In this way, the conductors, with their identification into the resources of the group, create the basis for the individual's belief in the group to be reawakened.

18.2 A Somewhat Groupless Image of Humanity

The beginnings of the dominance of an image of man oriented towards performance and interested in his personal advancement lie in Protestantism. Associated with the names of Calvin and Max Weber, the idea developed with the rise of industrialization and the emergence of the bourgeoisie that one had to earn God's favor and thus one's happiness in life through one's own performance and effort. Individuals had to do something meaningful in the eyes of society in order to stand before God, in other words, to "achieve something". Over time, and with the progression of capitalism, the mechanisms of discipline within the system and now self-discipline have become increasingly subtle (see Sloterdijk, 2009). Many people are now suffering from this, as the individual is often overwhelmed.

The Additional Benefit of Group Psychotherapy

Individual therapy can do a lot of good, but by its very nature, it lacks the group-related, sometimes the triangulating aspect. Here, the group also serves as a protection against abuse in the dyad (cf. Sect. 1.3.). The individual cannot solve problems that concern the group. The individual is sometimes merely the index patient or the delegated patient, the symptom bearer in a group (cf. Richter, 1975). Thus, the statements of individuals in the group can be interpreted as expressing the group dynamics or an important part of it. However, these interpretations also have a collectivizing, de-individualizing aspect, which should certainly have its place. This reflects a deep truth: that we are all unconsciously connected with others, for better or worse. This implies that defense needs can be satisfied in and with groups, but also that mental resources can be expressed.

All psychological experience is ultimately also a group phenomenon. This emphasis by the English author Dalal (1998) points out that we should question our categorization systems, especially as therapists. Central to psychological and psychotherapeutic thinking over the past hundred years has been the individual, the single person. We have learned to understand groups as a collection of individuals. However, we are still bound to the concept of individuals and cannot see that it is the group that shapes the identity of the individual, precedes it, and enables its specific role in society. Richter (2002) also critically reflected on this 40 years after his groundbreaking family-analytical work.

A Preliminary Conclusion

The first part of this book was intended to illustrate the deep anchoring of our group identity based on the socialization history of people in Western societies. It is difficult for us, including many highly decorated experts, and even one of the founders of group analysis, Foulkes, to consistently keep both in view: the group and the individual. Both create each other in a co-constructivist way, as was said in the intersubjectively influenced psychoanalysis about the transference-countertransference dynamics (cf. Jaenicke, 2006). It is not about the image of mutual influence, because this presupposes the existence of both sizes, the individual and the group. This shows that we had too limited assumptions about the functioning of our social systems and are now in the process of revising them.

Dalal does not deny that the personality of the individual is quite capable of influencing a group (cf. Dalal, 1998, p. 158). Rather, he wants to add the concept of the group in the individual to the widespread notion of the individual as part of a group, in order to more realistically depict and conceptualize the complex interplay of several perspectives on human psychological life. But he does not stop there, because this would again establish a hierarchy, this time one that would overemphasize the importance of the group. According to Dalal (1998), it is about the simultaneous consideration and pursuit of both lines in the formation of psychological structures. A major mistake, in his view, is also the confusion of external influencing factors and the social environment. The separation of external and internal factors is not helpful, as it represents an artificial separation of interacting aspects. In this respect, even the concept of separating an "outside" and an "inside" is misleading. I agree with this. Just as the perception of the seemingly objective external always depends on the inner world of the individual, so does its inner world develop depending on the conditions of the environment in which an individual grows up. Therefore, the question of the chicken and the egg is irrelevant.

Individual, Group, and Natural Environment

Charim (2023) attests that the narcissistic society leads to a dead end, as the constant navel-gazing and self-optimization increasingly distances one from the experience of being embedded in something greater, higher, nature. We encounter this concern also in the thoughts that psychologists have about the interaction between human behavior and the events in nature triggered by global warming (cf. Bronswijk and Hausmann, 2022). The call is for a relativizing self-examination and a look at the shadow aspects of growth and power agglomeration. In the best case, groups are not "echo chambers," like the communities on the internet that push each other. They promote developments away from self-reference, egoism, and narcissism. The experience in groups allows the perception of one's own possibilities, opportunities, resources, and limits. Such groups thus enable self-experience as a participant, as a part-owner, without having to be the sole focus. They show what can all be achieved, with and for others, without being able to achieve everything that individuals want. Group participation can therefore lead to more satisfaction. In this respect, groups also follow the tradition of humanism, as it is currently represented, for example, by Sarah Bakewell (2023). She says: "So one is not a separate entity floating around as an individual in space. Regardless of our origin, we all grow up in a network of other people around us, which enables us to become a more humane person, precisely because we are connected to the roots of our being as humans." (2023, min 8.20 ff.). Group psychotherapy and analysis make this fact visible and tangible and can make the resources of the psychological common ground usable for all of us.

References

Bakewell, Sarah (2023) Podcast Sternstunde Philosophie. https://www.srf.ch/play/tv/sternstunde-philosophie/video/sarah-bakewell---humanisten-leben-erfuellter?urn=urn:srf:video:123ff5e4-191a-46c6-b05d-d6b29e11d543. Abgerufen am 2.12.2023.

Bronswijk, K v, Hausmann, C M (2022) (Hrsg) Climate Emotions—Klimakrise und psychische Gesundheit. Psychosozial-Verlag, Gießen

Charim, I (2023) Wie narzisstisch ist unsere Gesellschaft? Podcast Sternstunde der Philosophie vom 14.1.2023, https://open.spotify.com/episode/3RdAZOJYIqOA0DVy7UZIJR?si=B9BF8C9B-B08B-4433-908D-F71B2FF58399&utm_source=system-ua-share&nd=1 (Stand: 17.09.2023)

Dalal, F (1998) Taking the group seriously. Jessica Kingsley Publishers, London

Jaenicke, C (2006) Das Risiko der Verbundenheit. Klett-Cotta, Stuttgart

Richter, H E (1975) Eltern, Kind und Neurose. Rowohlt, Hamburg

Richter, H E (2002) „Eltern, Kind und Neurose" 40 Jahre danach. In: Psychoanalytische Familientherapie—Zeitschrift für Paar-, Familien- und Sozialtherapie: Migration und Familie. Nr. 4, 3. Jg., 2002, Heft I
Sloterdijk, P (2009) Du musst dein Leben ändern. Suhrkamp, Frankfurt
Ullman, E (1997) Close to the machine. City Light Books, San Francisco
Ullman, E (2018) Life in a code. Picador, London

The manufacturer's authorised representative in the EU is Springer Nature Customer Service Centre GmbH, Europaplatz 3, 69115 Heidelberg, Germany. If you have any concerns regarding our products, please contact ProductSafety@springernature.com

Printed and bound by CPI Group (UK) Ltd, Croydon, CR0 4YY

23/09/2026

02221543-0006